Unmasked Threat: Head & Neck Cancer

Richard

First Printing, 2024

Contents

1

Introduction

Head and neck squamous cell carcinoma (HNSCC) encompasses malignancies localized in the head and neck region, e.g. oral cavity, parasanal sinuses, salivary glands, pharynx and larynx, being the ninth most common malignancy worldwide (Bray et al., 2018). Main risk factors for the development of HNSCC include tobacco consumption, alcohol abuse, as well as chronic infection with human papilloma virus (Gupta et al., 2016). A multidisciplinary approach is required for the treatment of HNSCC, with surgery as an option in early stages of the disease, whereas a tri-modality treatment consisting of surgery and/or radiotherapy and chemotherapy is used in advanced stages (Sanderson, 2002).

There are several challenges for radiotherapy in the head and neck region such as the large extension of the treatment area, including as target volumes the primary tumor and affected lymph nodes, the complex anatomy, which starts with a narrow neck region and ends with the wider area of the shoulders, and different tissue densities such as air, bones and soft tissue. Furthermore, sensitive organs at risk (OARs) such as spinal cord, salivary glands, swallowing muscles, oral mucosa and visual system, with low dose tolerances, must be considered and spared during treatment planning in order to prevent late tissue complications, which can influence the quality of life of the patient.

Radiotherapy techniques such as photon-based intensity modulated radiation therapy (IMRT) have shown the potential to deliver high doses to the tumor, while reducing the doses to the OARs (Bhide et al., 2012; Marta et al., 2014; Hawkins et al., 2018). Proton therapy (PT) is a promising advanced technique for the treatment of HNSCC, due to the physical characteristics of protons such as their finite range and Bragg peak, allowing a high-dose conformity and improved dose reduction to the surrounding healthy tissue compared to photon irradiation. Diverse studies have addressed the advantages of PT compared to IMRT, demonstrating high conformal dose distributions and improved normal tissue sparing, while delivering the same dose to the target volume (Cozzi et al., 2001;

Steneker et al., 2006; Mendenhall et al., 2011; Simone et al., 2011; van de Water et al., 2011; van der Laan et al., 2013; Jakobi et al., 2015a). The main advantage of HNSCC proton over photon therapy is the reduced dose deposited to the OARs, which can be translated into reduced late radiotherapy-related toxicities (Jakobi et al., 2015b; van Dijk et al., 2016; McKeever et al., 2016).

Due to the finite range of protons, they are more sensitive to uncertainties that might occur during the treatment course, as errors in patient setup and proton range calculation, resulting in a potential degradation of the delivered dose. The International Commission on Radiation Units and Measurements (ICRU) reports recommend to account for possible uncertainties during treatment by a margin expansion of the target volume (ICRU, 1993; ICRU, 1999; ICRU, 2007). This approach, while it is commonly used in photon treatments, might not be sufficient to account for uncertainties in proton therapy. Robust treatment planning approaches, which include these potential uncertainties directly into the plan optimization process, have shown superior plan robustness over plans with a simple target volume margin expansion in HNSCC cases (Liu et al., 2012; Liu et al., 2013a; Liu et al., 2013b; Li et al., 2015b; van Dijk et al., 2016; Stützer et al., 2017b). Besides uncertainties in patient setup and proton range, anatomical variations during the treatment course, such as non-rigid variations in patient positioning, patient weight changes, and tumor shrinking, can cause a degradation from the planned dose, as shown in geometrical margin-based proton treatments (Kraan et al., 2013; Góra et al., 2015; Müller et al., 2015; Thomson et al., 2015; Stützer et al., 2017a).

The aim of this book is the evaluation of robust treatment planning techniques in a commercial treatment planning system (TPS) for HNSCC cases, considering uncertainties in patient setup, proton range and anatomical variations during the treatment course. First, the principles of proton therapy (Chapter 2) and concepts of robust treatment planning and evaluation (Chapters 3 and 4) are reviewed. Second, margin-based and robustly optimized plans are compared in Chapter 5 for a cohort with target volumes of unilateral location. Differences in dose distributions, doses to target volumes and OARs, and the influence of anatomical variations during the treatment course are investigated. And last, complex bilateral target volumes are evaluated in Chapter 6, considering the influence of weekly anatomy variations, together with setup and range uncertainties. A robust treatment plan considering additionally potential anatomical variations in the plan optimization is proposed and compared to a classic robustly optimized approach.

2

Proton Therapy

Contents

Radiation therapy (RT) uses ionizing radiation, generally as part of cancer treatment, to control or eliminate malignant tumors. The final aim of RT is to deliver the prescribed dose to the tumor, while sparing the surrounding normal tissues. Research in physics has contributed directly and indirectly to radiation therapy over the past century. Only months after their discovery by Wilhelm Conrad Röntgen in 1895, X-rays were used to treat a patient with breast cancer (Grubbé, 1933; Lederman, 1981). At present, usually RT employs a beam of high energetic X-rays (described as *photon beam*) generated as Bremsstrahlung with an electron linear accelerator and directed towards the tumor. However, in the recent years alternatives such as proton therapy (PT) have shown to be promising in RT, offering several advantages compared to photons. The following chapter gives an overview of PT. Further details can be found in McDonald and Fitzek (2010), Paganetti (2012), Degiovanni and Amaldi (2015), and Lee et al. (2018).

2.1 Rationale for Proton Therapy

The advantages of PT with respect to conventional photon therapy were first outlined by Robert R. Wilson (1946). The potential of proton beams for medical purposes was described by making use of the finite range and the Bragg peak of proton beams for treating tumors. Due to the low entrance dose and reduced dose distal to the target, the integral dose to the normal tissues is reduced compared to photon therapy, as represented in Figure 2.1.

For treatment purposes, usually multiple proton beams with several energies are combined to generate a spread-out Bragg peak (SOBP), in order to obtain a homogeneous depth dose plateau over the target. Advanced techniques such as intensity modulated proton therapy (IMPT) are able to generate high dose gradients, using the whole advantage of protons for radiation treatment.

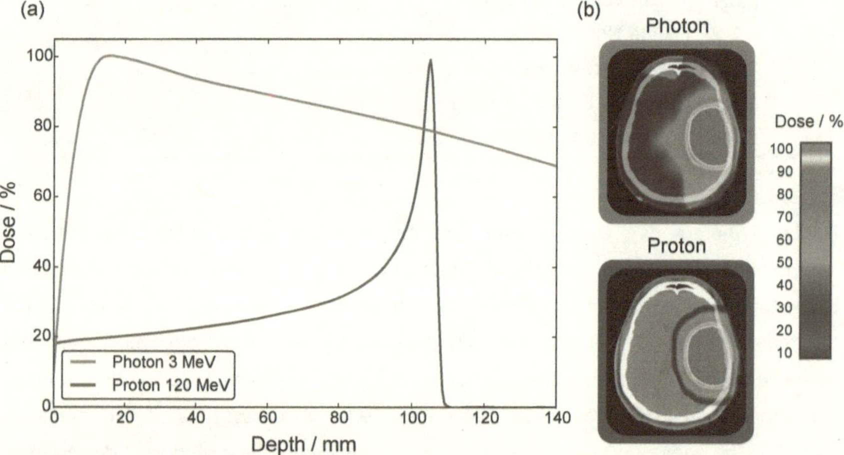

Figure 2.1. (a) Depth dose curves of monoenergetic photons (green) and protons (blue) in water, simulated with FLUKA 2011.2x.4 (Ferrari et al., 2005; Böhlen et al., 2014), courtesy of M.J. Gonzalez Torres. (b) Transversal computed tomography slices of the head (gray level) for a low grade glioma, overlaid with dose distributions in color wash. The target volume, to which the dose is prescribed, is contoured in cyan. The volume of surrounding normal tissue receiving low doses is much smaller for the proton plan (bottom) compared to the photon plan (top).

Assuming an identical target volume dose, proton therapy reduces the total energy deposited in the patient compared to photon therapy, which makes this technique attractive from a clinical point of view. High conformal doses in the target volume can be achieved with fewer fields. The superior properties of proton beams over photons can be translated into clinical benefit, firstly by an improved normal tissue sparing, while maintaining the dose to the tumor. In this case, the tumor control will be expected to be similar as with photons, whereas radiation-induced side effects will be reduced. This property is of particular interest for tumors located close to serially organized tissues such as spinal cord, brainstem or esophagus, where a small local overdose can cause significant complications. Moreover, in pediatric patients, the impact of the decreased integral dose and increased normal tissue sparing is even more significant, because of the reduced probability of secondary cancer induction (Miralbell et al., 2002; Paganetti and van Luijk, 2013). Secondly, protons allow dose escalation, which improves the local tumor control (Palm et al., 2019).

Although the dose distributions achievable with protons are superior to those achievable with photons, it is debatable whether the advantages of proton therapy are clinically relevant for all treatment sites (Ramaekers et al., 2011). Clinical evidence shows that protons (and other particles such as carbon ions) are superior to photon therapy in radioresistant tumors, which are close to organs at risk, such as chordoma, ocular melanoma, and pediatric tumors (Baumann et al., 2016; Lambrecht et al., 2018).

2.2 Beam Delivery Techniques

To generate a proton beam, the particles need to be accelerated to energies sufficient for treatment (approximately 220 MeV for 30 cm depth in water). Particle accelerators use an electric field to accelerate the protons. For PT, cyclical particle accelerators are required, in order to pass through the electric field several times until they reach sufficient energy for clinical application. The most common used devices for proton acceleration are cyclotrons and synchrotrons (Paganetti, 2012; Lee et al., 2018).

Cyclotrons accelerate protons within a fixed constant magnetic field. In a first step, low-energy protons are injected into the center of a disc-shaped accelerating cavity, gaining kinetic energy by passing through accelerating cavities within the disc. The constant magnetic field binds the protons to a circular path within the disc, but with each rotation they spiral radially outward increasing their energy. When the protons meet the most outer orbit, they are peeled off and directed to the beamline for clinical use. All protons leaving the cyclotron have the maximum available energy. To obtain lower energies, the beam is directed through low atomic number materials of variable thicknesses, which interact with the protons to lower their energy to the required energy for the patient treatment. The cyclotron delivers a nearly continuous output of protons.

Synchrotrons accelerate protons in a circular beamline with a fixed radius by boosting their energy in each revolution. During each rotation the magnetic field, which keep the protons constrained within the ring, must be synchronously increased to maintain a stable proton orbit. Once the protons reach the required energy for treatment, they are spilled into the beamline and directed to the treatment room by a series of focusing and bending magnets. Synchrotrons produce beams in a pulsed beam structure requiring a period to fill for acceleration and spill into the treatment room, typically taking 2-5 seconds per energy layer.

Once the protons have been accelerated, they are guided to the gantry for delivery to the patient. To shape the treatment field, two dose delivery techniques are currently applied in PT: passive scattering and pencil beam scanning.

2.2.1 Passive Scattering

Passive scattering uses the focused proton beam transported from the accelerator and scatters it through single or double scatterers in order to obtain a beam with large field size. At the same time, the beam energy is modulated to spread out the Bragg peaks location over the target volume in depth through a range modulator. The system is configured to produce a homogeneous dose distribution with the same penetration across the field. For clinical treatment, the beam is shaped by an aperture to match the lateral extension of the tumor and by a range compensator to conform the distal Bragg peaks to the distal surface of the target (Figure 2.2a).

A limitation of passive scattering is the fixed width of the SOBP over the lateral field extension, which can derive in a significant dose outside the target volume, typically proximal to the target since the range is adjusted through the compensator to match the distal target geometry.

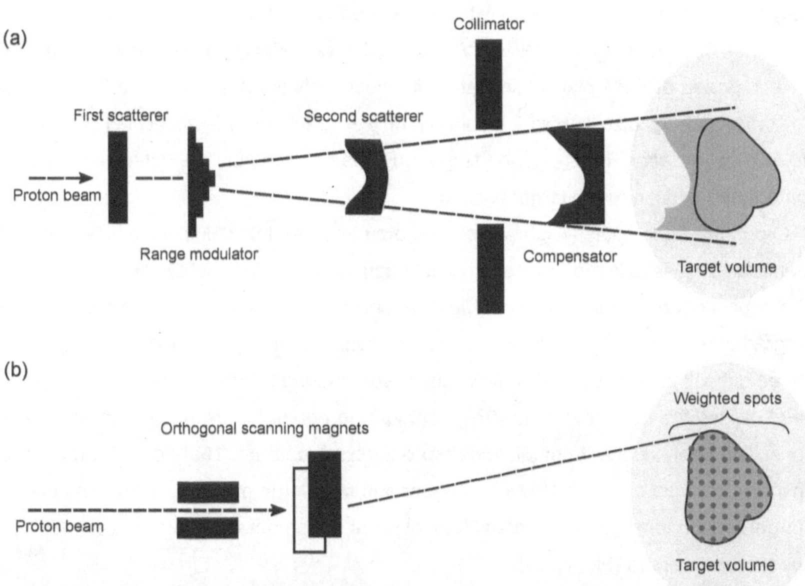

Figure 2.2. Scheme of a passive scattering system (a) and a pencil beam scanning system (b). The yellow and red color represent low dose and high dose regions, respectively. In passive scattering, the distal field edge is shaped by the range compensator to match the distal target geometry; however, in the proximal surface high dose regions may be present. Pencil beam scanning avoids this issue.

2.2.2 Pencil Beam Scanning

Pencil beam scanning (PBS) is gradually replacing passive scattering, and it was used for the treatment planning calculations in this book (Unkelbach and Paganetti, 2018). In this technique, two pairs of orthogonal dipole magnets are used to steer the unscattered proton beam to the lateral extent of the target volume, delivering the focused pencil beam to predetermined positions with a desire number of protons, i.e. spot weights. An energy selection system adjust the beam energy to achieve the desired range. The delivered dose is the superposition of each of the small pencil beam doses. No additional scattering or energy modulation devices are required (Figure 2.2b).

For PBS plan optimization, the TPS considers each pencil beam Bragg peak explicitly, specifying each treatment field as a list of Bragg peaks, each with a certain proton energy, the number of protons to be delivered and the lateral location of the Bragg peak. Two main categories of PBS plan optimization for dose delivery can be defined: *single-field optimization* (SFO), also known as delivery of a single-field uniform dose (SFUD), and *multi-field optimization* (MFO), depending of how the spot weights are optimized to ensure a homogeneous dose to the target volume.

SFO optimizes the spots weights of each proton treatment field, in such a way that a homogeneous dose is delivered to the target by each individual field. SFO can be considered as the equivalent of treating with open fields in photon therapy. This technique creates low dose gradients, especially inside the target; however, because of its limited modulation, it might be difficult to achieve sufficient normal tissue sparing (Figure 2.3a).

MFO utilizes the flexibility of the PBS technique to create highly modulated dose distributions. The spot weights from all fields are optimized together. Therefore, the dose from each individual field can be highly inhomogeneous, with large gradients inside and outside the target. The inhomogeneous doses from all fields are summed up to achieve a homogeneous target coverage (Figure 2.3b).

(a) Single-field optimization (SFO)

Field 1 Field 2 Sum

Dose / %

30 40 50 60 70 80 90 100 110

Field 1 Field 2 Sum

(b) Multi-field optimization (MFO)

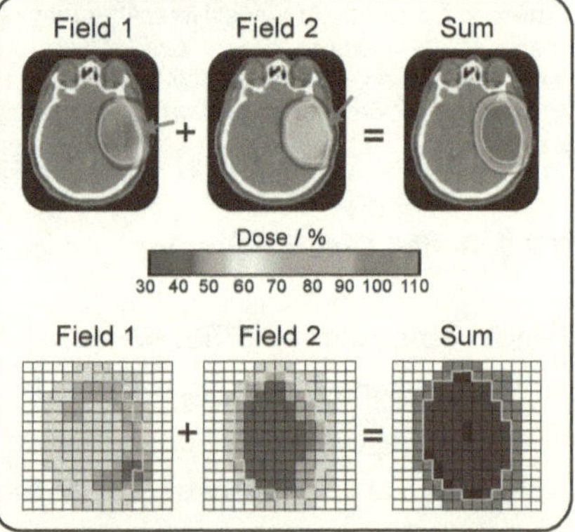

Figure 2.3. Exemplary patient (top) and schematic representation (bottom) of single-field optimization (a), where each treatment field delivers an homogeneous dose to the target, and multi-field optimization (b), where the dose from each field to the target can be highly inhomogeneous due to its high modulation. In both examples the target volume is delineated in cyan, and the field direction is indicated by a red arrow.

2.3 Uncertainties in Proton Therapy

Due to their physical characteristics, i.e. the finite range in tissue and the sensitivity to differences in tissue density, proton fields are more sensitive to uncertainties than photon fields used in conventional X-ray based radiotherapy. The different uncertainties might induce a shift of the Bragg peak location with respect to the planned location, with the potential consequence of not only degrading the dose to the tumor, but overdosaging the surrounding normal tissue and critical organs at risk. An overview of different sources of uncertainty in PT are discussed in the following.

2.3.1 Target Volume Definition

The ICRU provided in its reports 50 and 62 (ICRU, 1993; ICRU, 1999) the framework for prescribing, recording and reporting doses in RT, specifically in photon therapy, whereas the report 78 addresses the dose prescription and reporting in proton therapy (ICRU, 2007). For this effect, different target volumes are defined (Figure 2.4):

- *Gross tumor volume* (GTV). The GTV corresponds to the gross palpable or visible, demonstrable extent and location of the malignant growth. It may consist of primary tumor, metastatic lymphadenopathy, or other metastases. If the tumor has been removed, e.g. by previous surgery, no GTV can be defined.
- *Clinical target volume* (CTV). The CTV is a tissue volume containing a demonstrable GTV and/or subclinical malignant disease, that must be treated adequately in order to achieve the aim of radiotherapy. In cases where the initial GTV was surgically removed, the tumor bed is typically considered as a CTV.
- *Planning target volume* (PTV). The PTV is a geometrical concept used for treatment planning, defined to select an appropriate field configuration to ensure that the prescribed dose is actually delivered to the CTV. The PTV is conventionally used for dose prescription and dose reporting.

The target volume definition is linked with uncertainty (Unkelbach et al., 2018). The GTV definition is limited to the image resolution and the visualization of surrogates of the tumor instead of actual tumor cells. The delineation of the CTV also has uncertainty because the current medical image modalities cannot visualize microscopical subclinical disease (Apolle et al., 2017). The PTV concept relies on the static dose cloud approximation, i.e. the

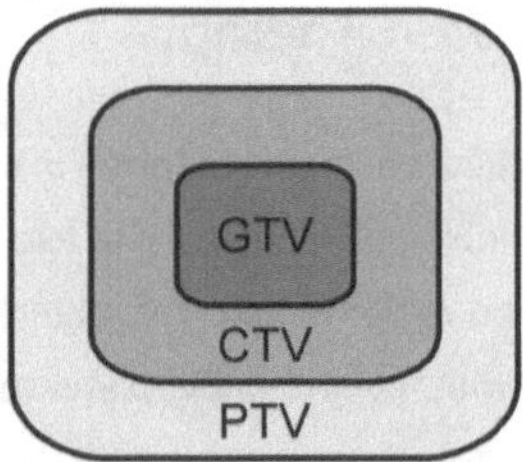

Figure 2.4. Target volume definition according to ICRU 50 and 62.

assumption that the CTV will receive the prescribed dose as long as it stays within the PTV. While this assumption works in general for photon therapy, where the PTV concept is widely used in clinical practice, there are several limitations when it is applied to proton therapy. In some cases, independent of the CTV-to-PTV margin expansion, the PTV concept does not guarantee an adequate CTV coverage in proton therapy.

2.3.2 Range Uncertainty

For the generation of treatment plans, a planning computed tomography (CT) of the patient is used as standard for plan optimization in RT. The information of the linear X-ray attenuation coefficients is converted into CT numbers, which can be translated with the electron density of the tissue. In proton therapy, the CT number is converted to stopping power ratio (SPR) for the calculation of the dose distribution. SPR values depend on the physical density, elemental composition and mean excitation energy of the material. For practical purposes, the correlation between CT number and SPR can be established for example through a stoichiometric model, which is clinically accepted (Schneider et al., 1996). New methods such as dual-energy CT-based SPR prediction have been studied in the last years, and will contribute to more accurate proton range predictions (Möhler et al., 2016; Wohlfahrt et al., 2017; Möhler et al., 2018).

Tissue density heterogeneities also add uncertainty to the range prediction. The delivered dose distribution will be sensitive to the exact position of the heterogeneities traversed by the proton beam. For instance, if the density heterogeneity is shifted in relation to the field, e.g. due to a misalignment or motion of the patient, the Bragg peaks will be shifted in depth, as displayed in Figure 2.5, which may lead to dose distortion and degradation in the target volume with respect to the predicted dose distribution (Lomax, 2008a).

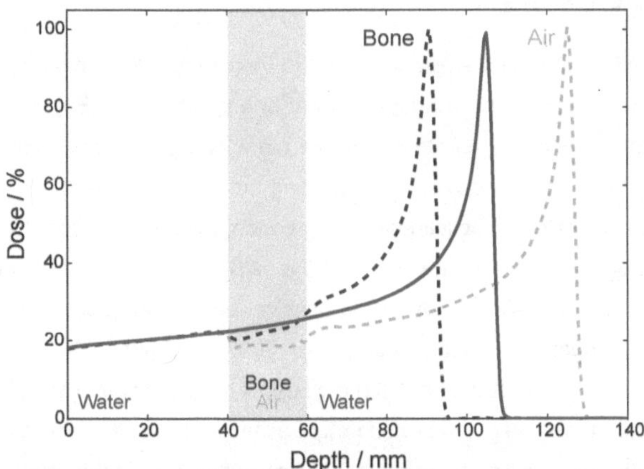

Figure 2.5. Proton range uncertainty to tissue density heterogeneities. The blue curve represents a Bragg peak of a 120 MeV proton beam in water, without heterogeneities. Tissue heterogeneities in the beam path (light red) decrease (e.g. bone, in brown) or increase (e.g. air, in orange) the proton range, leading to a shift of the Bragg peak. Depth dose curves were simulated with FLUKA 2011.2x.4 (Ferrari et al., 2005; Böhlen et al., 2014), courtesy of M.J. Gonzalez Torres.

2.3.3 Setup Uncertainty

A setup error is usually defined as a rigid shift of the patient with respect to the planned position relative to the isocenter (Unkelbach et al., 2018). The setup error has two components: a systematic component, defined as a mean shift displacement with respect to the planned position, and a random component, which considers variations between treatment fractions around the mean shift. It is expected for the systematic setup error to be close or equal to zero, and the random setup error to be small.

The impact of setup errors on the dose distribution can be more detrimental in proton therapy than in photon therapy: a patient shift might lead to misalignment of tissue heterogeneities in the beam entrance path and thereby causes degradation of the Bragg peak. Furthermore, the setup error has a different impact on each treatment field, and might lead to a misalignment of the individual field dose contributions. Therefore, setup errors do not simply lead to a lateral shift of the dose distribution, but may severely degrade it (Lomax, 2008b; Liebl et al., 2014; Unkelbach et al., 2018). Improved immobilization devices and image guidance are considered in PT to reduce the setup uncertainty during the treatment.

2.3.4 Biological Uncertainty

The biological effect of radiotherapy is related to the energy deposition of the beam in a cellular level. Proton beams have a higher linear energy transfer (LET) in the Bragg peak region compared to photons, i.e. they transfer more energy to the tissue per unit track length, causing more cellular damage. To account for the biological effect of the radiation type, the relative biological effectiveness (RBE) concept was proposed. It is assumed that the RBE value for protons is a constant, with the value of 1.1 recommended as a clinical appropriated value, i.e. 10% less of proton physical dose is needed to deliver the same biological effect compared to photon dose (ICRU, 2007; Paganetti, 2018)

Recent *in vitro* experiments suggest that the RBE is not a constant value, but it increases to values over 1.1 at the end of the proton range, being related to the increase of the LET at the distal edge of the Bragg peak. Further research is focused on the modeling of variable RBE values *in vitro* and *in vivo*, as well as biological plan optimization based on RBE and LET uncertainties (Paganetti, 2014; Jones, 2017; Lühr et al., 2018; Bai et al., 2019; Eulitz et al., 2019).

2.3.5 Anatomical Variations

Anatomical uncertainties might have an important impact on the delivered fraction dose, resulting in insufficient tumor coverage and/or overdosage of critical healthy structures, due to the tissue changes along the proton beam path. Random anatomical changes, such as variations in cavity filling, e.g. nasal cavity, bowel and bladder, organ motion and non-rigid shifts in patient positioning such as changes in the shoulder position, mandible and neck flexion, might be present between fractions and cause a degradation in the planned dose.

Conversely, systematic gradual anatomical variations can arise during the treatment course, such as patient weight gain or loss and tumor shrinkage. Dose degradation due to systematic treatment-induced anatomical variations in proton therapy is well documented in the literature. For instance, for head and neck cases, Kraan et al. (2013) showed a reduction of the target coverage and increase in hotspots for oropharyngeal tumors when recalculating the planned dose to a control CT acquired during the treatment course, whereas Stützer et al. (2017a) found in a patient cohort with head and neck cancer similar results regarding target coverage degradation and hotspots in a CT acquired about 4 weeks after the treatment beginning. Furthermore, van de Water et al. (2018) reported that variations in the nasal cavity filling during the treatment course may also degrade the planned dose distribution in SFO plans. In other body regions, Szeto et al. (2016) found target coverage degradation and increase in the dose to organs at risk for lung tumors.

To assure the consistence of a proton plan over the course of the treatment, additional image guidance plays an important role in order to detect early anatomical variations that might lead to severe deviations to the planned dose, which might be an indication for plan adaptation, i.e. the calculation of a new treatment plan considering the new patient anatomy. Moreover, range verification methods show to be promising in detecting variations of the proton range during the treatment due to variations in the anatomy (Richter et al., 2016; Parodi and Polf, 2018).

3

Robust Treatment Planning and Robustness Evaluation

Contents

Due to the different uncertainties in proton therapy, discussed in the previous chapter, the delivered dose of a proton plan can vary greatly from the planned dose. The classic PTV concept, used extensively in photon therapy, may not be sufficient to account for uncertainties in PT plans. An optimal treatment plan needs to be *robust*, i.e. designed in such a way that deviations from the planned dose due to uncertainties during treatment delivery will not affect the quality of the treatment outcome.

Approaches to Achieve Plan Robustness

Uncertainties in proton therapy and their influence in treatment planning are known by clinical practitioners. To reduce the influence of such uncertainties in the planned dose, different pragmatic approaches have been employed. For instance, in the passive scattering technique, the setup uncertainty can be accounted for by the size of the collimator, whereas the range uncertainty can be accounted for by the compensator (ICRU, 2007; Paganetti,

2012). In PBS treatment planning, additional approaches may be used to achieve plan robustness.

Selection of treatment field angle and direction The angle and direction of the treatment fields must be chosen in such a way to avoid areas of large tissue heterogeneities along the beam path, as well as changes between density interfaces, e.g. air or bone with soft tissue. Moreover, regions where potential anatomical variations can be present should also be avoided (Casares-Magaz et al., 2014; Gorgisyan et al., 2017; Gravgaard Andersen et al., 2017; Unkelbach and Paganetti, 2018).

Treatment field-specific PTV Instead of applying an isotropic PTV to CTV margin expansion, field-specific margins can be used (Park et al., 2012). For each treatment field, a specific PTV margin can be created to account for the different uncertainties in setup and range around the CTV. The generation of treatment field-specific PTV margins is currently available in the commercial TPS Eclipse (Varian Medical Systems, Palo Alto, CA).

Single-field optimization As described in Section 2.2.2, in SFO uniform dose distributions in the target volume are generated by optimizing individually the spot weights of each treatment field, resulting in more robust plans compared to high modulated fields generated by the MFO approach. However, the SFO technique offers reduced organ at risk (OAR) sparing, especially for complex shaped target volumes.

3.1 Robust Treatment Planning

Instead of using margins or approaches as SFO, uncertainties can be accounted by *robust treatment planning*, also known as robust optimization (RO). In simple words, RO methods incorporate uncertainties directly into the plan optimization, resulting in treatment plans with improved plan quality and robustness (Liu et al., 2012; Li et al., 2015b; Unkelbach and Paganetti, 2018). Usually the uncertainties considered in the optimization are setup and range errors, although additional uncertainties such as anatomical variations might be also accounted for.

To understand the concept of RO in the plan optimization process, first the nominal plan optimization, without including uncertainties, will be defined as a mathematical problem, according to Unkelbach et al. (2018). A treatment planning goal, for instance a minimum dose to be delivered to the target volume or dose restrictions to the OARs, can be described by an objective function f, which is a function of the dose distribution d. An optimal treatment plan corresponds to a small value of f; therefore, in the plan optimization process the objective function f is minimized:

$$\begin{aligned} \underset{x}{\text{minimize}} \quad & f(d(x)) \\ \text{subject to} \quad & x \geq 0\,, \end{aligned} \tag{3.1}$$

where x correspond to the spot weights in proton therapy.

3.1.1 Including Uncertainties in the Optimization

The different uncertainties in the dose distribution can be accounted by error scenarios k, corresponding, for example, to combinations of patient setup errors, proton range errors, and anatomical variations from patient CT datasets. Each error scenario is associated with a dose distribution d^k, which likewise corresponds to an objective function value $f^k = f(d^k)$. A treatment plan will be *robust* if the dose distribution d^k is optimal for the majority of error scenarios k that may occur, i.e. if the value of f remains small. To translate this concept into mathematical terms, two main RO approaches have been defined:

- Stochastic programming (Unkelbach et al., 2009).
- Minimax optimization (Fredriksson et al., 2011).

Stochastic Programming

In stochastic programming, introduced by Unkelbach et al. (2009), all the possible error scenarios k are considered in the optimization. For each error scenario, an importance weight p_k is assigned, describing the probability that the determined scenario occurs. High weight is given to most likely to occur scenarios, whereas small weight is given to unlikely scenarios. The sum of the objective functions f evaluated for all error scenarios is minimized:

$$\underset{x}{\text{minimize}} \quad \sum_k p_k f(d^k(x))\,. \tag{3.2}$$

This approach, also referred to as *probabilistic approach*, aims to find a treatment plan that delivers an optimal dose distribution d^k for all error scenarios considered.

Minimax Optimization

In minimax optimization, introduced by Fredriksson et al. (2011), the worst-case scenario is considered in the plan optimization, defined as the scenario k in which the objective function f attains its highest value. The goal is to obtain a treatment plan which is optimal for the worst-case scenario; thus, the maximum value of f is minimized:

$$\underset{x}{\text{minimize}} \quad \max_{k} \left[f(d^k(x)) \right] . \tag{3.3}$$

In contrast to stochastic programming, no importance weights are considered, since the objective function is minimized with respect to the worst-case scenario. This approach is also referred to as the *worst-case approach*.

Some variations of the minimax approach have been additionally studied:

Composite worst-case Equation 3.3 considers one objective function. In reality, one might have a set of objective functions f_s for determined structures s (target volumes and OARs) with defined weighting factors w_s, which describe the relative importance of the objective. Thus, (3.3) can be rewritten as:

$$\underset{x}{\text{minimize}} \quad \max_{k} \sum_{s} w_s f_s(d^k(x)) . \tag{3.4}$$

In summary, the weighted sum of the objective functions f_s in the worst-case scenario is minimized. This generalization can be referred to as the *composite worst-case.*

Objective-wise worst-case A variation of the composite worst-case is the objective-wise worst-case, introduced by Chen et al. (2012). In this approach, the maximum of each objective function f_s over error scenarios k is considered individually:

$$\underset{x}{\text{minimize}} \quad \sum_{s} w_s \max_{k} \left[f_s(d_s^k(x)) \right] . \tag{3.5}$$

Each error scenario k can affect different objectives, i.e. one error scenario which leads to the worst-case of a objective f_{s1} might not be the same which leads to the worst case of the objective f_{s2}. This method was evaluated for multicriteria optimization and additional details can be found in Chen et al. (2012).

Voxel-wise worst-case The previously described worst-case approaches minimize only physically realizable scenarios, i.e. the doses on each voxel i contained in the structure s come from the same error scenario. A more conservative approach considers the contribution of each voxel i to the dose distribution d. Thus, the objective function f can then be defined as a sum of different contributions f_i from individual voxels i. The maximum over the scenarios for each voxel separately is minimized:

$$\underset{x}{\text{minimize}} \quad \sum_s w_s \sum_i \max_k \left[f_i(d_i^k(x)) \right] . \tag{3.6}$$

This optimization approach is known as voxel-wise worst-case, and it was first introduced by Pflugfelder et al. (2008).

3.1.2 Differences Between Approaches

The described RO methods applied to IMPT treatment planning result in superior robustness against uncertainties, compared to the use of a simple PTV margin expansion. In general, there is no consensus whether one RO approach is superior to the others. However, depending of certain conditions, as geometry and planning objectives, some differences between approaches might appear.

If there are severe conflicts between different planning objectives, for instance due to the proximity of a dose limiting OAR to the CTV (e.g. salivary glands, pharyngeal muscles, visual system and spinal cord in head and neck cases), the composite worst-case approach may perform worse than the voxel-vise worst-case; however, both approaches perform better than the objective-wise worst-case (Fredriksson and Bokrantz, 2014). Conversely, minimax approaches are more robust in target doses compared to stochastic programming. Therefore, an explicit selection of the objectives f might be needed to preserve the overall plan robustness, as well as the specification of the relative importance w_s of each planning objective (Unkelbach et al., 2018).

Implementation in commercial TPS

Some of the RO approaches currently described are already implemented in different commercial TPS for clinical use. These algorithms are not only restricted to proton therapy, thus they might be applied as well for photon therapy planning:

- Composite worst-case: RayStation (RaySearch Laboratories AG, Stockholm, Sweden)
- Voxel-wise worst-case: Eclipse (Varian Medical Systems, Palo Alto, CA)
- Stochastic programming: Pinnacle^3 (Philips Radiation Oncology Systems, Fitchburg, WI)

In this book, RayStation was used for treatment planning. Uncertainty parameters that can be included in the optimization are setup uncertainties, defined as rigid patient isocenter shifts; range uncertainty, defined as an over- and undershoot of the nominal proton range; and anatomical variations, defined as different patient CT datasets, originally developed for 4D plan optimization. For the plan optimization, it is possible to combine nominal objectives (i.e. without considering uncertainties) with robust objectives for different structures, assigning determined importance weights.

3.2 Robustness Evaluation

More than 30 years ago, Goitein (1985) proposed that together with the evaluation of the nominal plan doses, an error analysis of the plans should be performed. For plan optimization in IMPT, this idea gains relevance due to the potential dose deviation that may occur due to uncertainties, as described in the previous chapter. Although robust optimized plans are designed to consider error scenarios into the plan optimization, it should be evaluated whether the planning goals are still fulfilled in presence of uncertainties.

The main idea consists on the plan recalculation considering different error scenarios, for example combinations of setup and range errors, defined as shifts of the patient isocenter and rescaling of the proton range (Langen and Zhu, 2018). These error scenario doses will be referred to as *perturbed dose distributions*. After the generation of perturbed dose distributions, the plan robustness against uncertainties can be evaluated by diverse methods.

3.2.1 Error Scenarios

Fixed Error Scenarios

To account for setup errors, a simple approach is to define rigid shifts in relation to the patient isocenter. The magnitude of the shift can be the same magnitude as used for the RO planning, or considering a defined confidence interval (Lomax et al., 2001; Albertini et al.,

2011; Liu et al., 2012; Trofimov et al., 2012; Liu et al., 2013b; Lowe et al., 2016). Modeling of range errors considers usually a minimum and maximum value, corresponding to the maximal expected under- and overshoot of the proton range, respectively. Further, perturbed dose distributions are calculated considering error scenarios with different realizations of setup and range errors.

The fixed perturbed error scenarios do not consider the effect of the fractionation and its influence on the plan robustness, especially in setup errors. In a typical fractionated treatment, daily random setup errors are present, due to changes in the patient positioning; thus, considering a setup error to be systematic might be an overconservative approach. However, such perturbed dose distributions may give a general overview of the plan robustness. To account for the effects of fractionation, Lowe et al. (2016) considered for the generation of perturbed dose distributions smaller confidence intervals as the used by Albertini et al. (2011).

Statistical Assessment

The effects of statistical uncertainties in the plan robustness can be quantified calculating a large number of perturbed dose distributions, also known as Monte Carlo sampling (Kraan et al., 2013; Park et al., 2013). Range errors are considered as systematic, whereas setup errors comprise a systematic and a random component. Systematic setup errors are considered equal for the whole treatment course, and random setup errors are sampled per fraction usually from a Gaussian distribution; thus, the influence of fractionated treatment on the total uncertainty can be assessed.

A Monte Carlo sampling of perturbed dose distributions gives more realistic results, since the resulting error scenario might be an actual outcome from a fractionated treatment. However, to achieve a sufficient accuracy, a large number of error scenarios need to be computed, which might be impractical in clinical practice.

Polynomial Chaos Expansion

The principle of polynomial chaos expansion (PCE) is to approximate the dose distribution as a polynomial function of the setup and range error. The PCE is constructed calculating first a limited number of perturbed dose distributions and fitting the results into polynomial functions. After post-processing, the resulting PCE function defines a model of the dose distribution as function of the error, allowing to calculate further perturbed dose distributions for new error scenarios in almost no time (Perkó et al., 2016).

One limitation is the computational cost required to generate the PCE, being over 60 minutes. Moreover, the PCE needs first to be generated for each patient, making this method difficult to use for the evaluation of plan robustness directly after the nominal plan optimization in clinical routine.

3.2.2 Visual Evaluation of Plan Robustness

After the calculation of perturbed dose distributions, the generated data needs to be evaluated. Different visual evaluation methods can be performed, in order to help with the decision whether a treatment plan is clinically acceptable, and if its robustness is still preserved in the perturbed scenarios. Different methods to visualize plan robustness are depicted in Figure 3.1 and discussed in the following.

Dose-Volume Histogram Bands

A visual representation in the patient dose-volume histogram (DVH) was proposed by Trofimov et al. (2012) in the form of DVH bands, which shows the variability of the treatment plan in presence of uncertainties. The band envelop is defined from the overall minimum and maximum dose values extracted from the previously calculated perturbed dose distributions in a determined volume structure. In general terms, a wide DVH band indicates a reduced plan robustness, i.e. the perturbed dose distribution can deviate greatly from the nominal dose, and vice versa.

Voxel-Wise Worst-Case Dose Distribution

A dose distribution can be generated considering, from the perturbed dose distributions, the minimum voxel value for voxels inside the target volume, and the maximum value for voxels outside the target (Lomax et al., 2001). The resulting worst-case dose distributions allows a direct visualization of regions where the target coverage might decrease, as well as overdosage of the OARs, when in presence of the considered uncertainties.

Error Bar Dose Distribution

Another approach to visualize the robustness of a treatment plan is by the generation of an error bar dose distribution, which represents the spread of dose values within the considered perturbed dose distributions (Albertini et al., 2011). Each error bar voxel value is calculated by considering the difference between the maximum and minimum value from the perturbed dose distributions in each voxel. Values near to zero, i.e. a small spread, indicate a high plan robustness. Furthermore, an error bar-volume histogram (EVH) can be generated in an analogous way as DVH for each structure, where the plan will be robust if the histogram line is closer to zero.

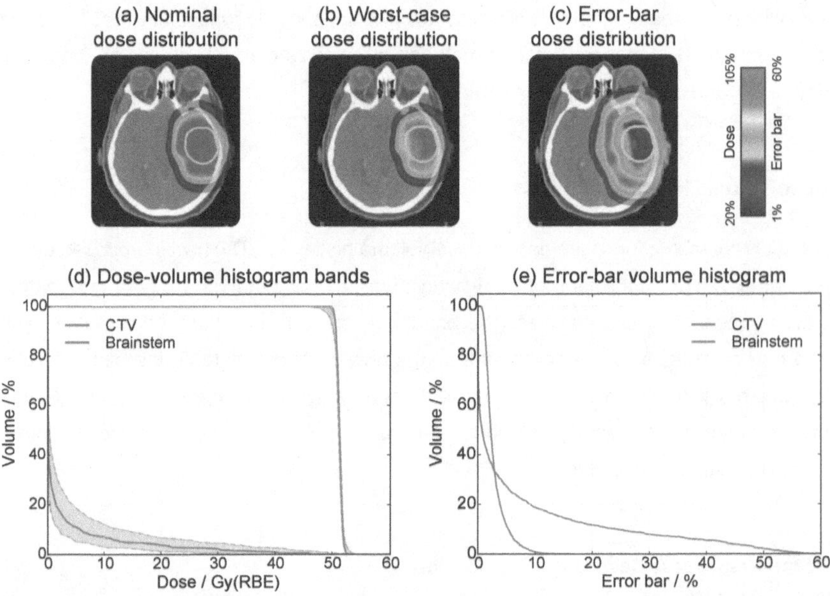

Figure 3.1. Representation of the diverse tools for visualizing plan robustness. The nominal dose distribution (a) can be compared with a voxel-wise worst-case dose distribution considering the overall minimum voxel value inside the CTV (b). An error-bar dose distribution (c) can be generated considering the difference between the maximum and minimum voxel values from the perturbed dose distributions. The envelope of perturbed dose distributions can be visualized as dose-volume histogram bands (d), and from the error-bar dose distribution an error bar-volume histogram can be generated (e).

3.2.3 Summary

Diverse methods to evaluate the robustness of a treatment plan are available. All methods rely on the calculation of perturbed dose distributions considering different error scenarios, evaluating how the calculated treatment plan behaves in the presence of uncertainties. Although there is no consensus about the selection of error scenarios for evaluation, robustness analysis provides in general additional information, which can be use for clinical decision making between two treatment plans. Some of the mentioned methods, such as the visualization of DVH bands and worst-case dose distributions, have been recently incorporated in commercial TPSs.

4

Illustration of Robust Treatment Planning in a Simple Geometry

Contents

In the following chapter, robust treatment planning together with a simplified robustness evaluation will be illustrated for a simple anatomy geometry in a cohort of low grade glioma patients. The region surrounding the target volume in brain tumors consists of mostly homogeneous brain tissue. Moreover, there are typically no severe anatomical variations during a fractionated treatment course. Setup errors are small due to the stable location inside the skull, the use of a thermoplastic mask for fixation, and image-guide positioning.

Robust treatment plans, using the CTV as target volume and defining setup and range errors for the plan optimization are calculated. Afterward, a simplified robustness evaluation is performed, with the generation of perturbed dose distributions considering fixed variations in the setup error together with systematic random errors.

4.1 Plan Design

Patient Data and Dose Prescription

A cohort consisting of ten low grade glioma patients was selected, extracted from a larger cohort originally recruited for a multicentric *in silico* study comparing different radiation treatment modalities for low grade gliomas (Eekers et al., 2018). Each patient dataset consisted of a planning CT, with the GTV delineated by an expert radiation oncologist. The CTV was defined as the GTV plus 1 cm margin. Several OARs in the brain region were further contoured.

The prescribed dose to the CTV was 50.4 Gy(RBE) in 28 fractions, with defined clinical objectives:

- the minimum dose to the 98% fo the target volume should be at least 95% of the prescribed dose ($D_{98\%} \geq 95\%$, near minimum dose),
- the maximum dose to the 2% of the target volume should be less than or equal to the 107% of the prescribed dose ($D_{2\%} \leq 107\%$, near maximum dose), and
- the volume of the CTV receiving 95% of the prescribed dose should be at least 99% ($V_{95\%} \geq 99\%$).

OARs with defined dose limits were: brain ($D_{2\%} < 60$ Gy,), brainstem ($D_{2\%} < 54$ Gy) and optic chiasm ($D_{2\%} < 55$ Gy). Additional organs at risk were optimized to receive doses as low as possible.

Plan Optimization

The plans were generated and calculated using RayStation, research version 4.99. Defined TPS calculation parameters were used in this and the next chapters:

- pencil beam algorithm including heterogeneity corrections for plan calculation
- constant RBE of 1.1 for proton beams, as recommended by ICRU 78 (ICRU, 2007),
- dose calculation grid of $3 \times 3 \times 3$ mm^3,
- IBA universal nozzle, with a pencil beam sigma ranging from 8 mm (100 MeV) to 4 mm (220 MeV), where the spot distance and energy layer distance were calculated automatically by the TPS,
- for each treatment field, a range shifter of 7.5 cm water equivalent thickness was considered to allow dose deposition in shallow parts of the tumor, and

- robust optimization based on composite minimax approach.

Two treatment fields were used in the evaluated cases, with an air gap of 2 cm between patient surface and range shifter. For the minimax optimization, the robustness parameters were set to 2 mm for setup error in cardinal directions and 3.5% for range error, considering in total 21 scenarios for the plan optimization. Only objective functions related to the CTV were selected as robust.

Plan Robustness Evaluation

The robustness of the plans against setup and range uncertainties was evaluated by generating perturbed dose distributions with fixed setup and range errors, in a similar way as proposed by Albertini et al. (2011). First, setup errors were modeled by shifting the patient isocenter by 2, 3 or 4 mm along each major axes (x, y, z) and diagonal directions, in both positive and negative directions. Three samples of 14 dose distributions with each setup shift combination were generated, as depicted in Figure 4.1.

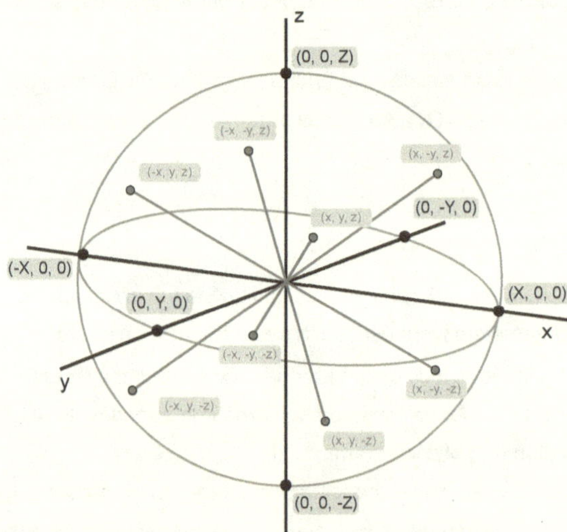

Figure 4.1. Selection of isocenter positions for the calculation of perturbed dose distirbutions. Maximum isocenter shifts are applied in the main axes directions X, Y, Z, whereas diagonal shifts corresponds to values of (x, y ,z) which value summed in quadrature corresponds to the maximum shift. Adapted from Albertini et al. (2011).

To assess the range error, for each setup shift, 42 perturbed dose distributions were generated: 14 without range error, 14 with a range error of 3.5% and 14 with a range error of -3.5%, resulting in overall 126 perturbed dose distributions per patient.

Dose statistics for the CTV coverage and OARs were extracted from each nominal and perturbed dose distributions. The worst-case value was extracted, defined as the minimum value for CTV coverage ($D_{98\%}$ and $V_{95\%}$ parameters), and the maximum value for CTV $D_{2\%}$ and OARs dose parameters. For each setup shift length (2, 3 and 4 mm), the worst-case values were extracted first from the perturbed dose distributions without range error (14 perturbed dose distributions), and second with range of $\pm$3.5% (26 perturbed dose distributions), to evaluate the influence of each error source. In total for each patient, 6 sets of worst-case doses were extracted and analyzed.

Furthermore, DVH bands as proposed by Trofimov et al. (2012) were generated for one exemplary patient considering, for each setup error, the band for the perturbed dose distributions without range error and range error of $\pm$3.5% separately.

4.2 Plan Results

4.2.1 Doses on Nominal Plan

Dose statistics for the nominal doses are summarized in Table 4.1. The nominal plan coverage of the CTV was fulfilled in all cases, with median (range) values for the $D_{98\%}$ of 99.6% (99.4–99.8%), whereas the volume receiving 95% of the prescribed dose ($V_{95\%}$) was 100% for all cases. The near maximum doses $D_{2\%}$ were below the objective of 107% of the prescribed dose, with median (range) values of 104.9% (103.7–106.1%). Regarding the OARs, the doses were below the dose limits in all cases.

4.2.2 Influence of Uncertainties in Plan Robustness

Influence of Setup Error in Plan Robustness

For each set of perturbed doses with defined setup error value (2, 3 and 4 mm), the worst-case values showed a decrease in the median CTV $D_{98\%}$ value of 2 percentage points from the nominal dose value. However, for all setup errors the CTV coverage fulfilled the planning objective ($D_{98\%} \geq 95\%$). The $V_{95\%}$ parameter was above 99% for setup errors of

Table 4.1. Nominal and worst-case dose statistics for each perturbed dose distribution set; median (range) of the ten patients.

ROI Metric	Nominal dose		Setup error	Worst-case dose Range 0%		Worst-case dose Range ±3.5%	
CTV $D_{98\%}$ (%)	99.6	(99.4–99.8)	2 mm	99.2	(98.9–99.5)	99.1	(98.4–99.3)
			3 mm	98.8	(98.1–99.2)	98.7	(97.6–99.1)
			4 mm	97.4	(96.7–98.5)	97.2	(96.5–97.2)
CTV $V_{95\%}$ (%)	100	(100–100)	2 mm	100	(99.9–100)	99.9	(99.9–100)
			3 mm	99.8	(99.6–100)	99.7	(99.5–100)
			4 mm	99.2	(98.8–99.8)	99.2	(98.5–99.7)
CTV $D_{2\%}$ (%)	104.9	(103.7–106.1)	2 mm	105.0	(103.9–106.3)	105.2	(103.9–106.3)
			3 mm	105.0	(104.0–106.3)	105.2	(104.0–106.3)
			4 mm	105.0	(104.0–106.3)	105.2	(104.0–106.4)
Brain $D_{2\%}$ (Gy)	52.2	(51.7–52.7)	2 mm	52.3	(51.8–52.8)	52.3	(51.8–52.8)
			3 mm	52.3	(51.8–52.8)	52.3	(51.8–52.8)
			4 mm	52.3	(51.8–52.8)	52.4	(51.8–52.8)
Brainstem $D_{2\%}$ (Gy)	50.8	(26.1–52.2)	2 mm	51.6	(29.0–52.4)	51.5	(32.3–52.7)
			3 mm	51.7	(30.4–52.9)	51.8	(33.6–52.8)
			4 mm	51.9	(31.9–53.2)	52.0	(34.9–52.9)
Optic chiasm $D_{2\%}$ (Gy)	50.0	(0.5–52.2)	2 mm	50.8	(0.9–52.4)	50.9	(1.9–52.8)
			3 mm	51.2	(1.0–52.5)	51.2	(2.2–52.9)
			4 mm	51.5	(1.2–52.8)	51.5	(2.4–53.1)

Abbreviations: ROI, region of interest; CTV, clinical target volume; $D_{98\%}$, dose to the 98% of the volume, $V_{95\%}$, volume receiving 95% of the prescribed dose, $D_{2\%}$, dose to the 2% of the volume.

2 and 3 mm, whereas one patient showed a value of 98.8% for setup error of 4 mm. High doses to the CTV ($D_{2\%}$) did not show major variations from the nominal dose in all cases.

Brain $D_{2\%}$ doses did not show variations for different setup errors, but a slight increase was observed in brainstem and optic chiasm $D_{2\%}$ doses with increasing setup error, yet the doses remained in acceptance levels.

Influence of Combined Setup and Range Error in Plan Robustness

When additionally range errors were considered, the median $D_{98\%}$ doses on the CTV showed a slight decrease up to 0.2 percentage points, but the target coverage fulfilling the clinical objective. The $V_{95\%}$ parameter showed no substantial differences from the per-

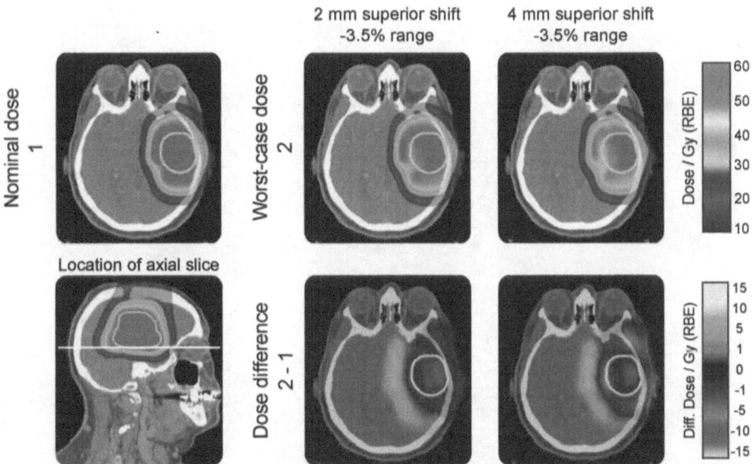

Figure 4.2. Dose distributions of nominal and worst-case doses for an exemplary patient, with the CTV delineated in cyan. The nominal dose (1) is compared with the worst-case dose distributions (2) for two realizations of setup errors (2 and 4 mm), showing a slight reduction in the CTV coverage, without compromising the clinical objective.

turbed dose distributions without range error. Regarding OARs, worst-case $D_{2\%}$ doses for brain, brainstem and chiasm showed no large variations from the situation without range error.

Dose statistics for the sets of perturbed dose distributions are summarized in Table 4.1. Dose distributions for an exemplary patient are depicted in Figure 4.2, and comparison of dose statistics and DVH bands for the same patient for CTV and OARs are depicted in Figures 4.3 and 4.4, respectively.

4.3 Discussion and Conclusion

In the present chapter, the application of minimax robust proton treatment planning has been illustrated in a simple geometry, by calculating robust plans with target volumes localized in the brain region for 10 cases and performing a simplified robustness analysis. The CTV coverage was preserved for different instances of setup and range errors, whereas the doses to the OARs remained below their dose limits.

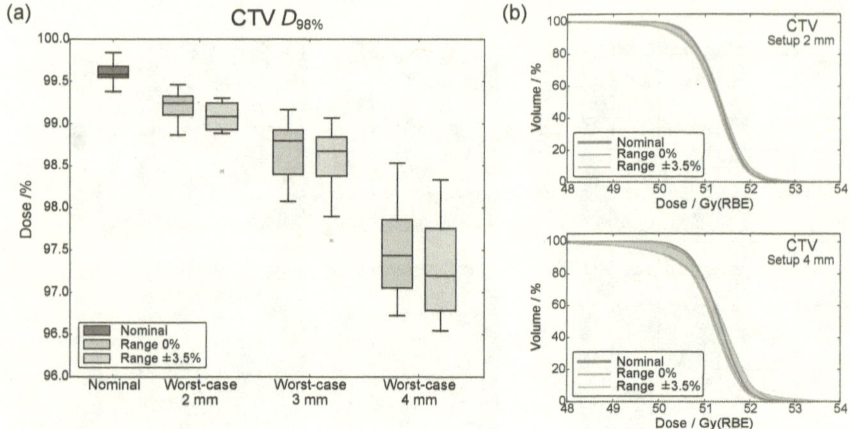

Figure 4.3. (a) Comparison of nominal and worst-case doses for the CTV $D_{98\%}$ parameter. Although the worst-case values are slightly smaller than the nominal dose, they still fulfill the planning objective of 95% of the prescribed dose. (b) DVH bands for an exemplary patient, considering the whole envelope of perturbed dose distributions for setup error of 2 mm (top) and 4 mm (bottom), for each range error. The bands for setup of 4 mm are wider, but fulfill the planning objective.

Evaluating both sources of uncertainty, setup errors played the most relevant role in CTV coverage degradation. Additional range errors did not show a large influence on the target coverage. The range error considered in the perturbed dose distributions was of the same magnitude as the range uncertainty considered in the plan optimization, therefore it is expected that the plans are robust against range errors of the same magnitude. The same was observed for the OAR doses, which did not show larger differences with and without range error in the worst-case dose; however, for the patient example in Figure 4.4, a wider DVH band is shown when the range error is taken into account for brainstem and optic chiasm. In this study, robust objective functions were considered only for the CTV. In principle, it is possible to apply robust functions also for the OARs, which might reduce the variation of the dose in the perturbed dose scenarios. Additional factors such as the objective function weighting and conflicting objectives between target volume and OARs must be considered.

Challenges of robust optimization in complex geometries In complex geometries such as head and neck squamous cell carcinoma (HNSCC), which is the main focus of this

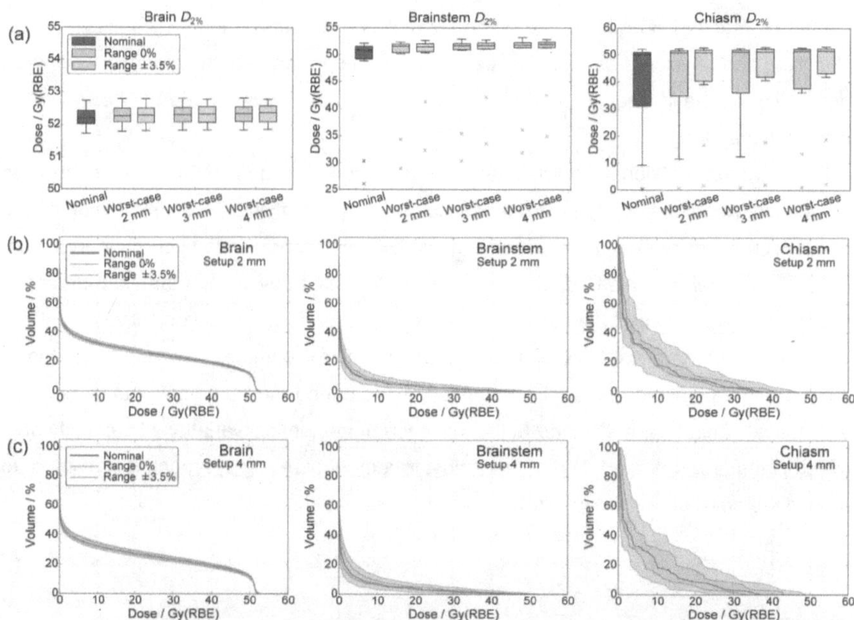

Figure 4.4. (a) Comparison of nominal and worst-case doses for the OARs $D_{2\%}$ parameter of all ten patients. (b) DVH bands for an exemplary patient, considering the whole envelope of perturbed dose distributions for setup error of 2 mm, for each range error. For brainstem and chiasm, the DVH band is wider when the range errors are considered. (c) DVH bands considering the perturbed dose distributions for setup errors of 4 mm.

book, usually two dose prescription levels for the CTV are defined. The low level covers the elective volume, whereas the high dose level considers the primary tumor and metastatic lymph nodes. Furthermore, several OARs with dose limits below the prescribed doses to the CTV are present, for instance spinal cord, salivary glands, oral mucosa, larynx and swallowing muscles. These OARs are relevant for important side effects such as myelitis, xerostomia, mucositis and dysphagia, which adds additional challenges to the robust plan optimization

In some HNSCC cases, the parotid glands might have portions bordering or overlapping with the CTV. For the planning objective definition, an auxiliary OAR planning volume, which considers only the portion outside the CTV, can be defined. By doing so, the CTV coverage will not be compromised; however, it might be possible that the desired sparing of the OAR cannot be reached, if an important portion of the volume is inside the CTV. In such cases, clinicians and physicists should discuss the relative importance of the planning objectives depending on the individual case, if more weight should be given to the CTV coverage or to the OAR sparing.

Furthermore, additional uncertainties should be considered in HNSCC cases, such as anatomical variations during the treatment course, as patient weight loss and tumor shrinkage, which might reduce the plan robustness. Different approaches such as in-treatment imaging together with plan adaptation are used, to detect deviations that might decrease the target coverage and/or increase the OAR dose beyond the clinical objectives.

In summary, there are additional challenges in RO for complex geometries related to the treatment planning and additional uncertainties during the treatment course, such as anatomical variations. In Chapter 6, the influence of anatomical variations in robustly optimized plans are evaluated, and a new robust treatment planning approach is proposed, to reduce the need of plan adaptation.

5

Evaluation of Robust Treatment Plans in Unilateral Head and Neck Squamous Cell Carcinoma

Contents

Unilateral head and neck irradiation is indicated for entities which present a reduced risk for contralateral spread, e.g. malignancies of major salivary glands, early-stage tonsil cancer, selected oral cavity cancer and in cases of re-irradiation (Leeman et al., 2017). Therefore, the target volume for radiation treatment may be confined to one side.

Several investigations have shown the potential of PT when irradiating unilateral HNSCC target volumes, regarding OAR sparing and reduction of the integral dose to the normal tissue. Passive scattering PT was compared against IMRT by Romesser et al. (2016), finding a significant normal tissue sparing with protons, which can be translated into reduced treatment toxicity. Regarding studies with PBS technique, Kandula et al. (2013) investigated differences between IMPT and IMRT dose distributions in a cohort of five unilateral HNSCC patients, finding similar results, with a substantial reduction in the integral dose when using protons. Furthermore, Zhu et al. (2014) investigated for one head and neck case the feasibility to include simultaneous integrated boost (SIB) within IMPT SFO planning, whereas

Stromberger et al. (2016) included a SIB with IMPT MFO planning for six unilateral HNSCC cases.

The mentioned studies have calculated the plans using a PTV margin expansion for the assessment of setup and range uncertainties in PT planning. However, robust optimization techniques have so far not been studied for unilateral HNSCC proton treatment. Conversely, no study has compared MFO and SFO in unilateral head and neck irradiation. Quan et al. (2013) compared both techniques in four bilateral HNSCC patients, finding higher robustness for the SFO plans, but with the price of higher parotid gland dose compared to MFO; however, this study did not consider robustly optimized plans.

The aims of the following *in silico* study are:

- to assess the feasibility of PBS proton therapy for unilateral head and neck squamous cell carcinoma (HNSCC),
- to compare IMPT single-field and multi-field optimization approaches, with either PTV-based optimization or CTV-based robust optimization and,
- to assess the robustness of the plans to uncertainties in patient setup, proton range and anatomical variations.

The work presented in this chapter has been published in Radiation Oncology and it was presented at the ESTRO 36 conference (Cubillos-Mesías et al., 2017a; Cubillos-Mesías et al., 2017b).

5.1 Study Design

5.1.1 Calculation Parameters

Patient Data

For the design of the planning study, eight patients treated with double scattering PT at the University Proton Therapy Dresden between March 2015 and June 2016 were selected. Inclusion criteria were the presence of delineated unilateral HNSCC volumes for treatment planning and a regular acquisition of control CTs (cCTs) during the treatment course, with an adequate length of the scanned field of view. The patient characteristics are presented in Table 5.1.

Each patient dataset consisted of a planning CT (pCT) and several cCTs (median: 6,

Table 5.1. Patient and tumor characteristics of the unilateral HNSCC cohort.

Patient	Primary tumor site	Gender	TNM-stage
1	Left parotid gland[1]	F	pT1 N0 M0
2	Right parotid gland[1]	M	pT1 N0 M0
3	Right minor salivary glands	M	pT1 N2b M0
4	Lateral border of tongue	F	pT1 N2b M0
5	Right tonsil	M	pT2 N2b M0
6	Maxillary sinus	M	rcT2 N1 M0
7	Left parotid gland[1]	M	pT4a N0 M0
8	Right submandibular gland	M	prT2 N0 M0

[1] Patients with ipsilateral parotid gland surgically removed due to pathology.

range: 3–13) acquired during the course of the treatment using an in-room dual energy CT on-rails (Siemens SOMATOM Definition AS, Siemens Healthineers, Forchheim, Germany).

Two CTV levels were considered for the planning study: a high-risk CTV which includes the primary tumor, surgical cavity and potential metastatic lymph nodes, and a low-risk CTV which includes the elective unilateral lymph nodes. Delineated OARs were spinal cord, brainstem, parotid glands, larynx, oral mucosa, pharyngeal constrictor muscles and esophageal inlet muscle, as depicted in Figure 5.1. The volumes were contoured on the pCT by an experienced radiation oncologist. In three patients the ipsilateral parotid gland was surgically removed due to pathology.

Each cCT was at first registered to the pCT by rigid image registration with focus on the bony region. Following manual corrections if necessary, a deformable image registration (DIR) between both datasets was performed (Weistrand and Svensson, 2014). After the registrations were available, the contoured volumes on the pCT were transferred to each cCT, being subsequently reviewed and corrected by the same radiation oncologist.

Treatment Planning

Proton treatment plans were optimized and analyzed in the TPS RayStation, research version 4.99. Four PBS proton plans were generated for each patient:

- MFO_{PTV} – Conventional MFO plan, considering the PTV as target volume for treatment planning.
- SFO_{PTV} – Conventional SFO plan, considering the PTV as target volume for treat-

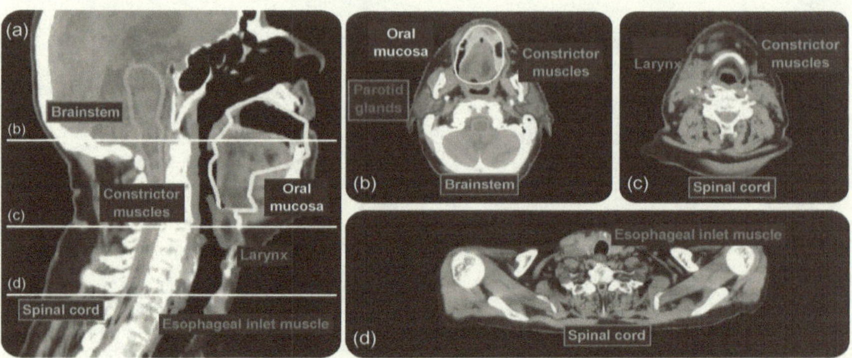

Figure 5.1. (a) Sagittal CT slice illustrating the delineated OARs. The OARs considered in the plan optimization are depicted by a red border. White lines represent the transversal slice locations in (b-d).

ment planning.

- MFO_{Rob} – Robustly optimized MFO plan, considering the CTV as target volume for treatment planning.
- SFO_{Rob} – Robustly optimized SFO plan, considering the CTV as target volume for treatment planning.

The robustly optimized plans were generated accounting for 3 mm setup errors and ±3.5% range errors. The robust optimization considers in total 21 scenarios combining setup and range errors. For the plan optimization, only objective functions related to the target volumes were selected as robust (Li et al., 2015b).

Each of the four plans per patient was generated using two or three treatment fields with the same gantry and couch angle configuration, as presented in Table 5.2, avoiding entering through risk structures and regions with high inhomogeneity gradients throughout the beam path. The dose distributions were calculated considering a constant relative biological effectiveness (RBE) of 1.1 for proton beams. Additional calculation parameters were set as described in Section 4.1, with an air gap between patient surface and range shifter of 3 cm.

The prescribed doses for the target volumes were 50.3 Gy(RBE) to the low-risk region and 68 Gy(RBE) to the high-risk region, delivered in 34 fractions. For the optimization of PTV-based plans, two PTVs were generated by isotropic expansion of each CTV by 5 mm.

Table 5.2. Treatment field gantry and couch angles used on the unilateral HNSCC plans per each patient.

	Field 1		Field 2		Field 3	
Patient	Gantry	Couch	Gantry	Couch	Gantry	Couch
1	30°	340°	80°	340°	–	–
2	320°	10°	280°	10°	–	–
3	340°	20°	280°	20°	–	–
4	345°	20°	290°	20°	–	–
5	340°	20°	280°	20°	190°	0°
6	340°	20°	280°	20°	200°	0°
7	30°	340°	80°	340°	–	–
8	345°	20°	290°	20°	–	–

The plans were calculated using a SIB. An additional transitional intermediate volume between low-risk and high-risk region of 10 mm margin was created to assure a steep SIB dose gradient (van der Voort et al., 2016).

The four plans were optimized to deliver the prescribed dose to the target volumes following the protocol at the University Proton Therapy Dresden, i.e. the minimum dose to the 98% of the target volume (near minimum dose) should be at least 95% of the prescribed dose ($D_{98\%} \geq 95\%$). Moreover, the dose to the 2% of the target volume (near maximum dose) should be less than 107% of the prescribed dose ($D_{2\%} \leq 107\%$). For PTV-based approaches, the PTV was selected as target volume for the optimization, whereas for robust optimized plan the CTV was selected. For evaluation purposes, the doses in the CTV in the four plans were considered.

The doses to the OARs were optimized as indicated in Table 5.3, considering the spinal cord, brainstem and parotid gland in the optimization. The remaining OARs were not considered in the plan optimization, but for dose reporting[1].

5.1.2 Plan Robustness Evaluation

Influence of Anatomical Variations

To evaluate the influence of anatomical variations in the planned dose distributions during the treatment course, each plan was recalculated on each available cCT, as an approxima-

[1]The remaining OARs were not available when the plans were optimized, but contoured afterwards.

Table 5.3. Treatment planning objectives for delineated volumes.

Structure	Planning objective	
CTV (PTV)[1]	$D_{98\%}$	$\geq$ 95% of prescribed dose
	$D_{2\%}$	$\leq$ 107% of prescribed dose
Spinal cord	D_{max}	< 45 Gy
Brainstem	D_{max}	< 54 Gy
Parotid gland	D_{median}	$\leq$ 26 Gy
Larynx	D_{mean}	No specified objective
Oral mucosa	D_{mean}	No specified objective
Pharyngeal constrictor muscles	D_{mean}	No specified objective
Esophageal inlet muscle	D_{mean}	No specified objective

[1] CTV or PTV as planning target structure depending of the plan approach.

tion of the dose delivered on a specific fraction. To evaluate and compare the approximate effective delivered dose within the whole treatment course with the nominal planned dose, total cumulative doses (D_{Cum}) were computed for each plan. Each recalculated dose on the cCT was deformed to the pCT and summed. This procedure, known as dose accumulation, was performed in RayStation using the DIR previously generated between pCT and cCTs. The workflow to generate total cumulative doses is depicted in Figure 5.2.

Influence of Setup and Range Uncertainties

As mentioned in Section 3.2.1, robustness evaluation considering fixed setup error values neglects the fractionation effect, i.e. the influence of interfractional random setup errors during the treatment course that reduce the total setup uncertainty due to the convergence of random errors. To evaluate the robustness considering a realistic clinical setting, a method similar as proposed by Park et al. (2013) was implemented.

The method consists of the calculation of integral-treatment perturbed doses considering random fraction-wise setup errors and systematic range errors. For each treatment fraction n, three random numbers were drawn from a Gaussian distribution with mean value $\mu = 0$ and standard deviation $\sigma = 2.5$ mm for the isocenter shift in the cardinal directions (x_n, y_n, z_n). Three fixed range error values of -3.5%, 0% and +3.5% were selected, considering the range errors as systematic, i.e. being the same for all fractions. For each range error value, 34 single-fraction doses, each with a different isocenter shift (i.e. random setup

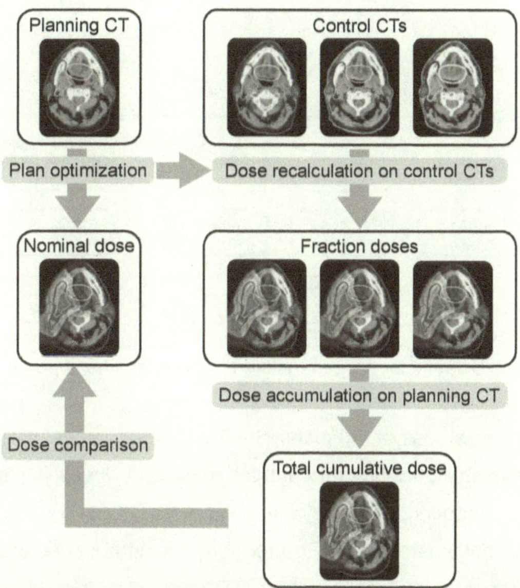

Figure 5.2. Workflow for the calculation of total cumulative doses D_{Cum}, recalculating the plan in each cCT and accumulating the dose in the planning CT.

error) were calculated, and posteriorly summed up to generate an integral-treatment perturbed dose, which considers the variations in the setup error per fraction. This procedure was repeated 10 times for each range error value, resulting in a set of 30 integral-treatment perturbed doses (Figure 5.3).

Two sets of integral-treatment perturbed doses were generated. For the first set, it was assumed that the anatomy of the pCT was maintained during the whole treatment course, hence the single-fraction doses were calculated considering the anatomy of the pCT. These integral-treatment perturbed doses are denominated as D_{PerNom}.

For the second set, the same procedure was repeated to evaluate the plan robustness considering additionally potential anatomical variations during the treatment course. Again, 30 integral-treatment perturbed doses were generated, considering the same random setup errors and range errors previously determined, but also considering the respective anatomy of the cCT for fraction dose calculation. These integral-treatment perturbed doses are denominated as D_{PerCum}.

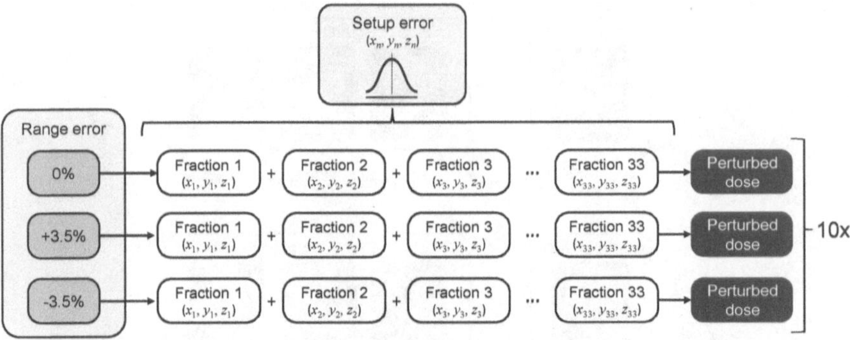

Figure 5.3. Scheme for the generation of integral-treatment perturbed doses.

To evaluate the robustness of the plans, the worst-case values of each dose parameter were extracted from the 30 integral-treatment perturbed doses per treatment plan. The worst-case value corresponds to the minimum value for CTV $D_{98\%}$ and maximum value for CTV $D_{2\%}$ and OAR dose parameters. Furthermore, the number of perturbed doses fulfilling the clinical objective of $D_{98\%} \geq 95\%$ for both CTVs was quantified. The total width, defined as the differences between maximum and minimum CTV $D_{98\%}$ value extracted from the set of 30 perturbed doses, was also calculated and compared between plans.

The calculation of both sets of integral-treatment of perturbed doses was efficiently implemented in RayStation via scripting, calculating in a step-wise basis perturbed fraction doses with random setup errors and systematic range errors, and dose accumulation considering the anatomy of either the pCT or cCT for the generation of integral-treatment perturbed doses. A summary of the abbreviations used for each evaluated set of dose distributions is described in Table 5.4.

Statistical Analysis

One-way analysis of variance (ANOVA) followed by post-hoc two-sample independent *t*-tests were performed in SPSS v.25 (IBM Corporation, Armonk, NY) to test significant differences in dose parameters between the four plans, including Bonferroni correction for multiple testing. Two-sided paired *t*-tests were used to determine significant differences between the nominal dose D_{Nom}, total cumulative doses D_{Cum}, and perturbed doses D_{PerNom} and D_{PerCum}. A p-value < 0.05 was considered to be significant.

Table 5.4. Nomenclature for evaluated dose distributions.

Dose name	Description
D_{Nom}	Nominal dose on pCT
D_{Cum}	Total cumulative dose, considering the anatomy of the cCTs
D_{PerNom}	Worst-case of integral-treatment perturbed dose considering anatomy of pCT
D_{PerCum}	Worst-case of integral-treatment perturbed dose considering anatomy of cCTs

5.2 Results

5.2.1 Evaluation of Nominal Plan Doses

Dose distributions for an exemplary patient are shown in Figure 5.4. For all patients, the CTV coverage was similar for the four plans, fulfilling the clinical objectives (median of $D_{98\%}$ values: 97.5–100.0% for the low-risk CTV, 98.5–99.8% for the hight-risk CTV), being slightly lower for the robust optimized plans, as shown in Figure 5.5. Only MFO_{Rob} plans showed a significantly lower $D_{98\%}$ dose for both low- and high-risk CTV, compared to the other plan approaches ($p \leq 0.04$). Regarding hot spots, $D_{2\%} \leq 107\%$ was met by the four plans in the high-risk CTV (median of $D_{2\%}$ values: 103.6–106.3%), but $D_{2\%}$ values higher than 107% were found in the low-risk CTV due to the dose gradient for the SIB treatment (median of $D_{2\%}$ values: 106.0–118.8%), with highest values for both PTV plan approaches, due to the margin expansion of the high-risk CTV used for the plan optimization.

The doses to the OARs were similar for all planning strategies. The near maximum doses to the spinal cord and brainstem D_{1cc} were far below the clinical constraints, with median D_{1cc} values of 1.8–2.0 Gy and 3.1–3.6 Gy, respectively. For the ipsilateral parotid gland, only contoured in five of the eight patients due to surgical removal in the others, high D_{median} values were found for both SFO_{PTV} and SFO_{Rob} plans (median D_{median} values of 30.3 and 28.5 Gy, respectively), with a significant increase for the SFO_{PTV} plan compared to the MFO_{PTV} and the MFO_{Rob} approaches ($p \leq 0.026$). The contralateral parotid gland was completely spared in all cases ($D_{median} \leq 0.1$ Gy), due to the target location and treatment field configuration, whereas the D_{mean} to larynx, oral mucosa, constrictor muscles and esophageal inlet muscle were similar for all plans, as shown in Figure 5.6. Detailed tabulated data can be found in the Appendix, Table A.2.

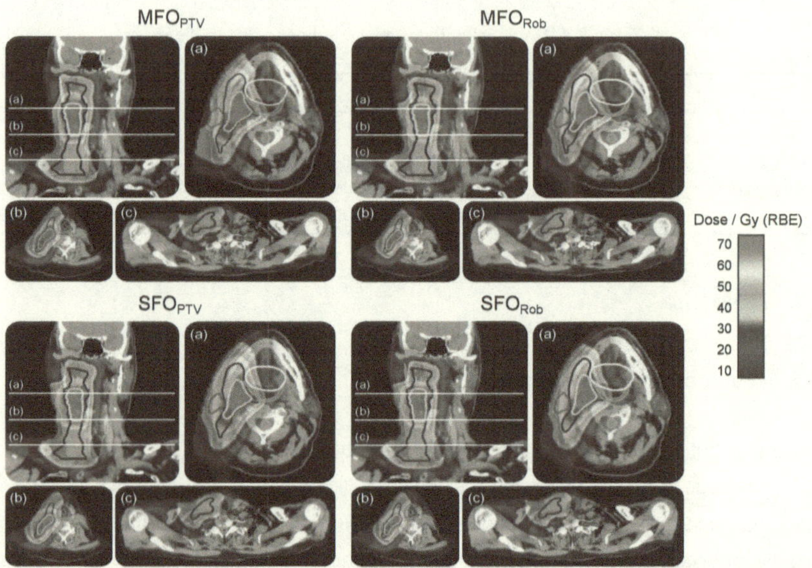

Figure 5.4. Dose distributions from MFO$_{PTV}$, MFO$_{Rob}$, SFO$_{PTV}$ and SFO$_{Rob}$ plans for an exemplary patient. White lines in the coronal view indicate the transversal slice position. Low-risk CTV and high-risk CTV are delineated in dark brown and pink, respectively. Both SFO approaches show higher doses to the ipsilateral parotid gland (delineated in purple), compared to the MFO plans.

5.2.2 Evaluation of Plan Robustness Against Uncertainties

Evaluation of Total Cumulative Doses

The $D_{98\%}$ values showed no significant statistical differences for the low- and high-risk CTV between nominal D_{Nom} and total cumulative doses D_{Cum} for the four plans. For one case, the high dose $D_{2\%}$ in the high-risk CTV was increased to 5.5% in the MFO$_{PTV}$ plan, whereas for another patient the $D_{98\%}$ on the high-risk CTV decreased to 94.8% in the MFO$_{Rob}$ plan, indicating that, even if the plans are robustly optimized, they might not be account for anatomical variations occurring during the treatment course.

Regarding the dose to the OARs, individual cases presented higher D_{Cum} doses compared to D_{Nom}, for example one patient showed an increase of 8 Gy in the larynx D_{mean} on both MFO$_{PTV}$ and SFO$_{PTV}$ plans. Spinal cord and brainstem D_{1cc} showed a slight median increase in the D_{Cum}, but remaining far below the dose constraints. The D_{median} values for ipsilateral parotid gland were slightly higher in the MFO_{PTV} plan (median increase of 2.4 Gy), but remaining higher for both SFO plans compared to both MFO approaches. However, the differences on the OAR doses between D_{Nom} and D_{Cum} were not significant for all four planning approaches.

The results for D_{Cum} for CTV $D_{98\%}$ and OAR dose statistics are shown in Figures 5.5 and 5.6. Detailed tabulated data can be found in the Appendix, Table A.2.

Evaluation of Robustness Against Uncertainties

Evaluation of D_{PerNom} doses The evaluation of the worst-case values from the set of integral-treatment perturbed doses considering the anatomy of the planning CT (D_{PerNom}) showed for the CTV doses no large variations between the four plans. No statistically significant differences were found in the low-risk CTV $D_{98\%}$ between D_{Nom} and D_{PerNom} doses in the four planning approaches, whereas a significant dose decrease in the high-risk CTV between the D_{Nom} and D_{PerNom} in the SFO_{Rob} approach was observed ($p = 0.043$). The other three plans showed no significant differences.

For individual cases, one patient showed a reduced $D_{98\%}$ value in low-risk CTV of 90.3% in the MFO_{PTV} plan, whereas for another patient a high-risk CTV $D_{98\%}$ value of 94.2% was found in the SFO_{Rob} approach. The other cases fulfilled the objective for both CTVs (Figure 5.5). Doses to the OARs showed a slight increase between D_{Nom} and D_{PerNom}, but without significant differences for all plans (Figure 5.6).

Evaluating the total set of 30 integral-treatment perturbed dose distributions, in general the majority fulfilled the clinical objective for both CTVs of $D_{98\%} > 95\%$, with a mean of 29.9 scenarios per plan (99.8%). In two cases, namely for MFO_{PTV} and SFO_{Rob} plans 2 and 4 scenarios were below the objective, respectively. The total width was typically largest for MFO_{PTV} plans (median (maximum) value of 1.8 (9.3) percentage points on the low-risk CTV), as shown in Figure 5.7. Detailed tabulated data can be found in the Appendix, Table A.1.

Evaluation of D_{PerCum} doses The worst-case values for the integral-treatment perturbed doses when anatomical variations during the treatment course are additionally accounted (D_{PerCum}) showed a dose reduction of both CTV $D_{98\%}$ dose parameters. The D_{PerCum} dose of the high-risk CTV $D_{98\%}$ was significantly reduced when compared to the D_{Cum} for MFO_{Rob} ($p = 0.019$) and SFO_{Rob} ($p = 0.041$) plans, whereas the PTV approaches showed

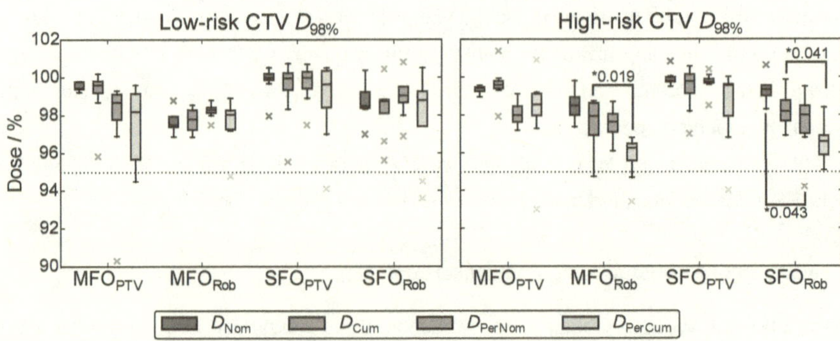

Figure 5.5. Comparison of the CTV $D_{98\%}$ between D_{Nom}, D_{Cum}, D_{PerNom} and D_{PerCum} for the whole unilateral patient cohort. Significant differences and p-values are indicated (*).

no significant differences (Figure 5.5). As in the previous evaluation, doses to the OARs showed a slight increase between D_{Cum} and D_{PerCum}, but without significant differences for all plans (Figure 5.6). Detailed tabulated data can be found in the Appendix, Table A.2.

For the set of 30 integral-treatment perturbed doses, the number of dose distributions fulfilling the clinical objective for both CTVs of $D_{98\%} > 95\%$ was also reduced compared to the D_{PerNom} set, with a minimum mean value of 26.8 scenarios (89.3%) in all planning approaches. The total width remained the largest for the MFO$_{PTV}$ approach (median (maximum) value of 1.9 (9.7) percentage points on the low-risk CTV), whereas the SFO$_{PTV}$ approach showed the smallest values (median (maximum) value of 0.7 (2.4) for the low-risk CTV). The variation in the total width from the D_{PerNom} doses was in general small, as shown in Figure 5.7. Detailed tabulated data can be found in the Appendix, Table A.1.

5.3 Discussion

In this study, four different PBS proton therapy approaches for HNSCC with unilateral target volumes, considering SFO and MFO with and without robust optimization, were compared. Furthermore, the influence of anatomical variations in the treatment course was evaluated, together with the robustness of the plans against random setup errors and systematic range errors.

Both PTV-based plan approaches showed small variations on the CTV coverage when

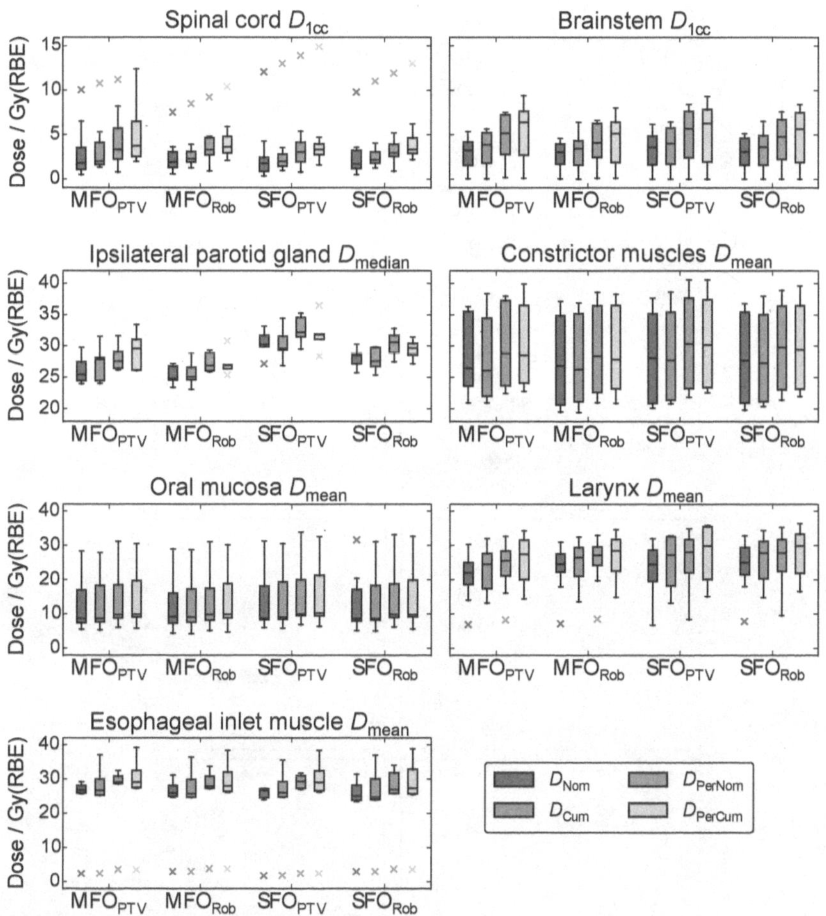

Figure 5.6. Comparison of OAR dose parameters between D_{Nom}, D_{Cum}, D_{PerNom} and D_{PerCum} for the whole unilateral patient cohort.

anatomical variations during the treatment course were considered (D_{Cum}), compared to the robustly optimized plans. Moreover, the MFO_{PTV} plan showed reduced robustness against additional setup and range errors, compared to the rest three approaches. Regarding OARs, both SFO plans delivered higher doses to the ipsilateral parotid gland, compared to the MFO plans.

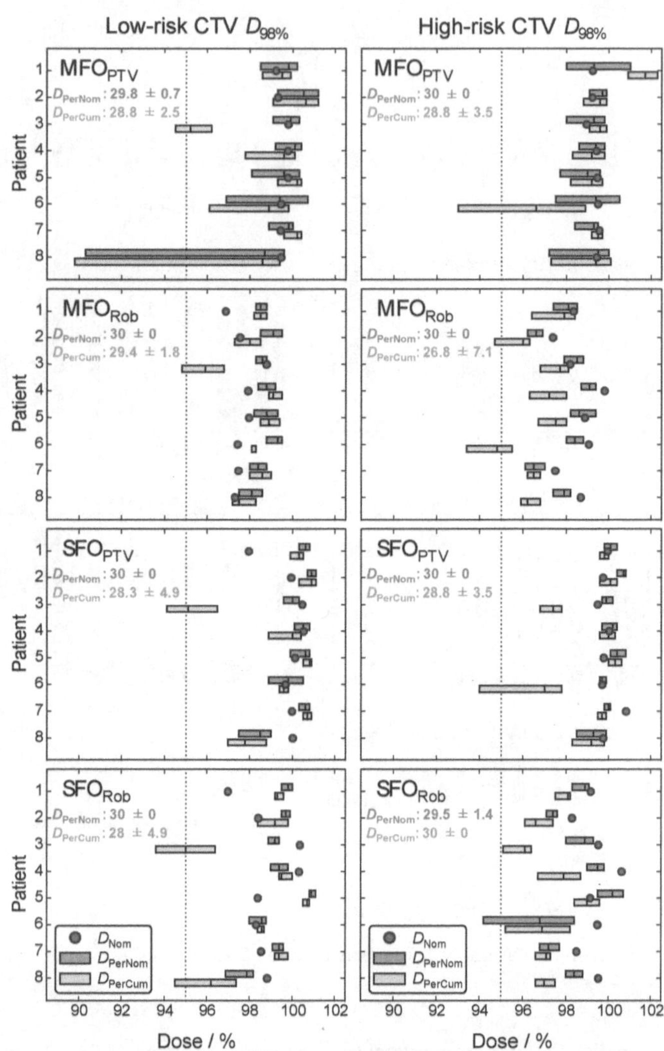

Figure 5.7. CTV $D_{98\%}$ statistics for the set of 30 integral-treatment perturbed doses and nominal plan values D_{Nom} per unilateral HNSCC plan and patient. The central line in each box represents the median value. The dashed lines represent the clinical objective (95%). The number of scenarios fulfilling the clinical objective are annotated for each approach (mean ± standard deviation).

Nominal plan doses Both PTV-based and robust optimized approaches fulfilled the target coverage requirements in the nominal plan. The near maximum doses to spinal cord and brainstem were far below the clinical constraints due to the unilateral target location, which allows for additional OAR sparing with proton fields. However, both SFO plans gave significantly higher D_{median} doses to the ipsilateral parotid gland compared to the MFO approaches, due to the reduced degrees of freedom in the field modulation and the resulting higher doses near the target volume (Figure 5.4). However, the chosen treatment configuration, with the proton fields entering through the tumor site, allowed to completely spare the contralateral parotid gland in all cases, with D_{median} doses near to zero, which helps to reduce the risk of secondary complications as severe xerostomia (Deasy et al., 2010).

The plan optimization did not have specific dose objectives to larynx, oral mucosa, constrictor muscles and esophageal inlet muscle, as these OARs were contoured afterwards, but the dose values were similar between the plan approaches, being the values close to or below the recommended D_{mean} constraints for reducing the risk of larynx edema and dysphagia (Rancati et al., 2010). Besides, the tumor size, which for unilateral irradiation is considerable smaller than bilateral targets, allows for an improved normal tissue sparing. It remains the question whether further OAR sparing is achievable if additional plan objectives for these organs were included.

For the PTV-based plans, a 5 mm margin expansion from the CTV was chosen, using the same values as used in photon therapy in Dresden. Romesser et al. (2016) and Stromberger et al. (2016) also used a 5 mm margin expansion in their studies, whereas Kandula et al. (2013) and Zhu et al. (2014) chose a 3 mm PTV margin. It has been investigated that PTV margins in photon planning should be calculated considering the systematic and random components of the setup errors, with margin recipes published (van Herk, 2004). However, the same principle cannot be easily translated into proton therapy, as the PTV concept might not account for such uncertainties.

For the robustly optimized plans, 3 mm for setup uncertainty and $\pm 3.5\%$ for range uncertainty were selected as robustness parameters. Van der Voort et al. (2016) investigated robustness recipes for IMPT plans for unilateral oropharyngeal cancer cases, determining a setup error value of 4.3 mm and a range error value of 3% to be used for the plan creation with their optimization algorithm. The proximity of the high-risk CTV to the edge of the low-risk CTV might increase the sensitivity to errors, therefore the recipe setup error value is higher as the one used in this study. However, the uncertainty values chosen are in agreement with the values from studies evaluating robust plans for bilateral HNSCC cases (Liu et al., 2013a; Liu et al., 2013b; Li et al., 2015b; van Dijk et al., 2016; Stützer et al., 2017b).

Plan robustness Analyzing the robustness of the plans, when first the anatomical variations during the treatment course were considered, the clinical objectives for CTV coverage and OAR sparing were fulfilled in most of the patients. For individual cases, a lower CTV dose than the planned dose could have been delivered to the CTV, for example one $\mathrm{MFO_{Rob}}$ case not fulfilling the coverage on the high-risk CTV. Anatomical variations during the treatment course can influence the cumulative dose distributions D_{Cum}, and even robustly optimized plans might not be sufficient to account for them.

Conversely, when different setup and range errors with a constant anatomy are considered, the four plans fulfilled in most of the cases the objective for target coverage, finding punctual cases when the dose might be reduced (cf. Figure 5.5). Although the majority of perturbed scenarios fulfilled the coverage of both CTVs, the total width was the largest for the $\mathrm{MFO_{PTV}}$ approach, indicating a reduced plan robustness against setup and range errors.

When additionally the anatomical variations in the cCTs were considered, the CTV $D_{98\%}$ doses were further reduced, even in robustly optimized approaches, being in line with the previous findings regarding total cumulative doses. Furthermore, the total width was the smallest for the $\mathrm{SFO_{PTV}}$ approach. Whereas plan robustness against setup and range uncertainties can be ensured when the anatomy of the planning CT is considered, the same cannot be affirmed when additionally anatomical variations are taken into account, since they were not considered as an additional source of uncertainty into the plan optimization. Thus, image guidance during proton therapy has special relevance in order to detect early changes in the anatomy that may lead to variations on the planned dose distributions which may be an indication for replanning. A new approach including information of anatomical variability in the plan optimization process will be proposed and evaluated on the next chapter.

Limitations of the study This study present some limitations. First, the size of the patient cohort was limited to the datasets available. At the time, the number of patients with unilateral HNSCC being treated with proton therapy in the institution was limited. Furthermore, the frequency of the acquisition of in-treatment cCTs was not consistent between patients, which may lead to uncertainties in the calculation of total cumulative doses.

Regarding the plan calculation parameters, PTV-based plans were calculated considering a CTV-to-PTV margin expansion of 5 mm. This value was larger than the setup error of 3 mm considered in robustly optimized plans, therefore an increased robustness might be expected for PTV-based plans. However, it was shown that independent of the planning approach, anatomy uncertainties during the treatment course, combined with setup and range errors, can decrease the plan robustness. Conversely, the robustness parameters selected for setup and range errors were chosen according to the literature, which is mostly published for bilateral targets. As mentioned before, a larger setup uncertainty might be considered in unilateral cases due to an increased sensitivity to errors, due to the size of the CTVs and the proximity of the high-risk CTV boundary to the low-risk CTV, which can influence the robustness of the plans against uncertainties, as well as the dose to the OARs (van der Voort et al., 2016).

Image artifacts, patient motion and differences in patient positioning between planning and control CT might derive in uncertainties in the image registration procedure and DIR, which can influence the contour propagation from planning to control CT, and the calculation of total cumulative doses (Brock et al., 2017; Paganelli et al., 2018; Ribeiro et al., 2018). To reduce the uncertainties in contouring, the radiation oncologist reviewed all contours propagated on each cCT. To reduce the uncertainties in image registration, an exact patient position between fractions is important, e.g. monitor the shoulder and mandible position for the head and neck region.

On the evaluation of robustness against uncertainties, for the generation of random setup errors, a sigma value of 2.5 mm was considered. Many studies have calculated the sigma for head and neck treatments in HNSCC for bilateral targets, with values near to 1.5 mm (van Kranen et al., 2009; Amelio et al., 2013; Ciardo et al., 2015; Lowe et al., 2016; Stützer et al., 2017b). The overconservative choice in the sigma value used in this study might result in fraction isocenter shifts values for x, y, z bigger than the 3 mm considered for the setup uncertainty in robust optimization, therefore the plan robustness might be decreased. This effect seems to be of importance when anatomical variations are considered, resulting in a summation of the error due to the isocenter setup and changes in anatomy. For bilateral HNSCC patient cases, studied in Chapter 6, a sigma of 1.5 mm for random setup errors is considered for the robustness evaluation.

The robustness analysis implemented by scripting in RayStation for the calculation of integral-treatment perturbed dose was intensively time-consuming within the used version of the TPS, making this method difficult to integrate in the clinical workflow for a prospective evaluation of plan robustness. Nowadays, additional tools for evaluation of the plan robustness are offered by commercial TPSs.

5.4 Conclusions

Four PBS proton therapy strategies were evaluated in a unilateral HNSCC cohort, showing adequate target coverage on the nominal plan, whereas the OAR dose remained similar between plans, with the exception of the ipsilateral parotid gland, where both SFO plan approaches showed higher D_{median} values compared to the MFO plans.

Both, PTV-based and robustly optimized plans, were sensitive to uncertainties in setup, range and anatomical variations for individual cases, leading to reduced target coverage and higher OAR doses. Hence, no plan strategy showed a decisive advantage regarding plan robustness and potential need of replanning.

6

Assessment of Anatomical Robustly Optimized Plans in Bilateral Head and Neck Squamous Cell Carcinoma

Contents

6.1 Anatomical Robust Optimization

The dosimetric advantages of proton therapy (PT) against photons for treatment of bilateral head and neck malignancies have been widely investigated in the last years, together with robustly optimized treatment approaches to account for uncertainties in patient setup and proton range, without the use of a PTV margin expansion (Liu et al., 2012; Li et al., 2015b; van Dijk et al., 2016; Stützer et al., 2017b).

Additional sources of uncertainty in PT for HNSCC are anatomical variations during the treatment course, for instance non-rigid variations in patient positioning, tumor shrinkage, and patient weight changes. Anatomic variations might cause a degradation of the planned dose, impacting the treatment plan quality, and requiring plan adaptation, as demonstrated for PTV-based IMPT plans (Kraan et al., 2013; Góra et al., 2015; Müller et al., 2015; Thomson et al., 2015; Stützer et al., 2017a). For robustly optimized plans, the impact of such anatomical variations in the dose distributions has not been investigated

Typically, the treatment plan optimization is based on one CT image dataset. 4D optimization techniques, including different CT phases, have been studied to account for respiratory motion in lung tumor cases (Li et al., 2015a; Liu et al., 2016; Engwall et al., 2018). Moreover, recent studies including additional CT datasets in the optimization have shown a higher robustness against anatomical variations during the treatment course, as Wang et al. (2017) for lung cases and van de Water et al. (2018) for sinonasal tumors.

For HNSCC cases, if additional information about potential anatomical variability could be included in the plan optimization, e.g. by additional CT image datasets, the plan robustness against anatomic variations might be increased, preserving the dose to the target volume, and therefore decreasing the need of plan adaptation.

In this study, a new robust treatment planning approach is proposed. The anatomical robustly optimized approach (aRO) considers additional effects of random non-rigid patient positioning variations in the plan optimization process, by the inclusion of additional CT datasets. The influence of diverse sources of uncertainty in the planned dose is further evaluated and compared with classical approaches.

The aims of the following *in silico* study are:

- to propose an anatomical robustly optimized plan approach which considers additionally non-rigid patient positioning variations in the plan optimization process,
- to compare the anatomical robustly optimized plan approach with a PTV-based approach and a classical robustly optimized approach (cRO) in terms of target coverage, dose to the OARs and integral dose to the healthy tissue,
- to quantify the influence of anatomical variations during the treatment course for anatomical, classical robustly optimized and PTV-based approaches,
- to quantify the influence of setup and range uncertainties together with anatomical variability for anatomical and classic robustly optimized plans, and

- to assess the need of plan adaptation of the proposed approach.

The work presented in this chapter has been published in Radiotherapy and Oncology and presented at ESTRO 37 and 38 conferences (Cubillos-Mesías et al., 2018; Cubillos-Mesías et al., 2019a; Cubillos-Mesías et al., 2019b).

6.2 Study Design

6.2.1 Calculation Parameters

Patient Data

The patient cohort for this study consisted of 20 patients with locoregionally advanced HNSCC treated at the University Hospital Dresden between August 2015 and July 2016. 17 patients were treated with IMRT, 2 with double scattered proton therapy and 1 with a mixed IMRT-proton treatment. Each patient dataset consisted of a planning CT acquired prior to treatment, and weekly scheduled control CTs (cCTs) acquired during the course of the treatment. A median number of 6 cCTs were acquired per patient (range: 4–7). Patient and tumor characteristics are listed in Table 6.1

Table 6.1. Patient and tumor characteristics of the bilateral HNSCC cohort.

Patient and tumor characteristics		Number
Gender	Female	2
	Male	18
Primary tumor site	Hypopharynx	3
	Oropharynx	8
	Oral cavity	8
	Larynx	1
Tumor classification	cT1	2
	cT2	3
	cT3	6
	cT4	9
Lymph node classification	cN0	2
	cN2	15
	cN3	3

The target volume consisted of two CTV levels: a high-risk CTV, including the primary tumor, surgical cavity and potential metastatic lymph nodes, and a low-risk CTV including the high-risk CTV and the elective bilateral lymph nodes. Considered critical OAR structures were spinal cord, brainstem, parotid glands, larynx, oral mucosa, pharyngeal constrictor muscles and esophageal inlet muscle (cf. Figure 5.1). CTVs and OARs were delineated on the planning CT by an experienced radiation oncologist. Each planning CT was registered with the weekly cCTs and the volumes were transferred and further reviewed, following the same procedure as described in Section 5.1.1.

Treatment Planning

Proton treatment plans were generated and analyzed in RayStation, research version 5.99. For each patient, three plans were calculated:

- Conventional PTV-based plan (PTVb), considering a CTV-to-PTV isotropic margin expansion of 5 mm, the PTVs as target volumes and the planning CT in the optimization.
- Classical robustly optimized plan (cRO), considering the CTVs as target volumes and the planning CT in the optimization.
- The proposed anatomical robustly optimized plan (aRO), considering the CTVs as target volumes and including additionally to the planning CT the first two (weekly) cCTs in the optimization, representing non-rigid patient positioning variations.

In this work, 3 mm for setup error and $\pm$3.5% for range error were selected as robustness parameters. For the aRO plans, since two additional CTs are included in the optimization, the algorithm considers a total of $3\times21=63$ different scenarios. For both, cRO and aRO plans, objective functions related to the target volumes, spinal cord, brainstem and parotid glands were selected as robust.

The prescribed doses to the target volumes were 57 Gy(RBE) to the low-risk CTV and 70 Gy(RBE) to the high-risk CTV, delivered with a SIB in 33 fractions. To assure a steep SIB dose gradient, an intermediate volume of 10 mm between both CTVs was generated (van der Voort et al., 2016; Stützer et al., 2017b). The doses to the CTVs were optimized following the institutional protocol: the minimum dose to the 98% of the CTV should be at least 95% of the prescribed dose ($D_{98\%} \geq 95\%$), and the dose to the 2% of the CTV should be less than 107% of the prescribed dose ($D_{2\%} \leq 107\%$). The doses to the OARs were

Table 6.2. Treatment planning objectives for delineated volumes.

Structure	Planning objective	
CTV (PTV)[1]	$D_{98\%}$	$\geq 95\%$
	$D_{2\%}$	$\leq 107\%$
Spinal cord	D_{max}	< 45 Gy
Brainstem	D_{max}	< 54 Gy
Parotid gland	D_{mean}	≤ 26 Gy
Larynx	D_{mean}	< 40 Gy
Oral mucosa	D_{mean}	As low as reasonable achievable
Pharyngeal constrictor muscles	D_{mean}	< 42 Gy
Esophageal inlet muscle	D_{mean}	As low as reasonable achievable

[1] CTV used in robust plans, PTV used in PTV-based plan

optimized following the institutional protocol and international recommendations, as listed in Table 6.2. The OAR portions outside the CTVs were considered in the optimization, to avoid conflicting objectives and to ensure an adequate CTV dose.

Each plan per patient was generated using three proton fields with the same configuration, with gantry angles of 180°, 60° and 300°, i.e. a posterior field and two anterior oblique fields, respectively. Additional calculation parameters were set as described in Section 4.1, with an air gap between patient surface and range shifter set to 3 cm.

6.2.2 Assessment of Plan Robustness

Influence of Anatomical Variations During Treatment Course

The influence of anatomical variations during the treatment course on the planned dose distribution was evaluated with a comprehensive method simulating an actual realistic treatment delivery.

First, weekly dose tracking was performed. This procedure consisted of the recalculation of the plan in each cCT, followed by the assessment of weekly cumulative doses, i.e. the dose delivered to the patient until the correspondent week considering the anatomical variations of each cCT, by non-rigidly deforming the recalculated dose to the planning CT for dose accumulation by DIR. Second, a total cumulative dose (D_{Cum}) was calculated, which simulates the treatment delivery by assessing the anatomy variations in the weekly cCTs during the whole treatment course, as depicted in Figure 6.1.

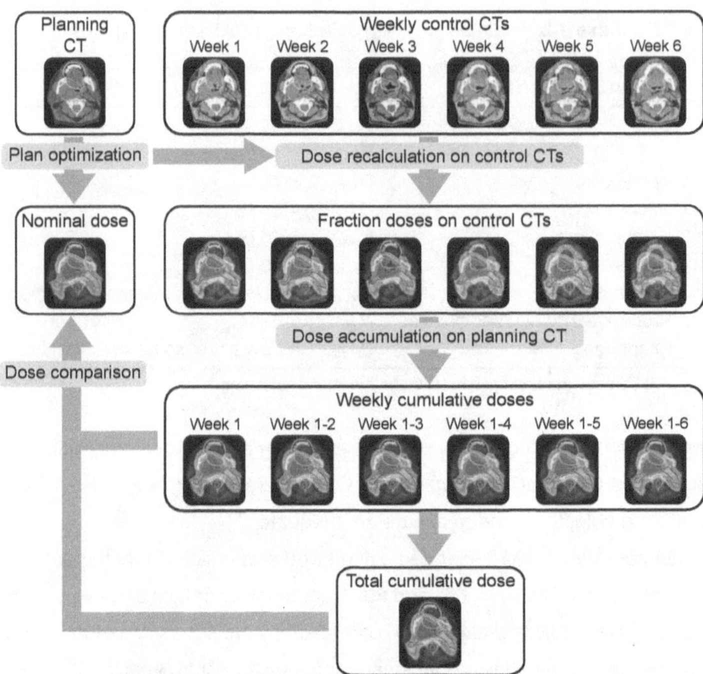

Figure 6.1. Workflow for weekly dose tracking and total dose accumulation. Weekly cumulative doses are generated from the recalculation of the nominal plan on each weekly cCT, and dose accumulation on the planning CT. Finally, a total cumulative dose simulates a complete treatment delivery.

The weekly and total cumulative doses were compared to the nominal plans (D_{Nom}) to evaluate the differences between the planned and the simulated delivered dose due to variations in the patient anatomy. For the target volume, the $D_{98\%}$ parameter was analyzed. The intervention criterion for plan adaptation was defined as a reduction in the target coverage below 95% of the prescribed dose.

Influence of Additional Setup and Range Uncertainties

The plan robustness, considering additionally uncertainties in setup and range, was evaluated for both robustly optimized approaches (cRO and aRO), following the method introduced in Section 5.1.2, cf. Figure 5.3. In this case the anatomy of the weekly cCTs was considered for the generation of 30 cumulative perturbed dose distributions per plan approach. Moreover, a more realistic standard deviation value of $\sigma = 1.5$ mm was selected for the generation of fraction random setup errors.

For evaluation purposes, the calculated set of 30 integral-treatment perturbed dose distributions were divided into two groups: perturbed doses with range error of 0% (D_{Per0}) and perturbed doses with range error of $\pm 3.5\%$ (D_{PerR}), corresponding to 10 and 20 cumulative perturbed dose distributions per treatment plan, respectively. Since the calculated perturbed dose distributions simulate a realistic fractionated treatment, the worst-case value of analyzed dose parameters was extracted for each group, corresponding to the minimum value for the CTV $D_{98\%}$ and the maximum value for the CTV $D_{2\%}$ and the OAR DVH parameters. The worst-case values were compared with the values from the nominal dose D_{Nom} and total cumulative doses D_{Cum}, to evaluate the influence on the plan robustness of:

(1) Anatomical variations alone (D_{Cum}).

(2) Anatomical variations plus random setup errors (D_{Per0}).

(3) Anatomical variations plus setup and range errors (D_{PerR}).

Moreover, the variation of dose parameters from the set of 30 integral-treatment perturbed dose distributions per plan, i.e. the total width defined as the difference between the maximum and minimum value for the corresponding dose statistic, was calculated and compared between the plans. A small width indicates a low variation between values, and therefore a higher robustness.

The calculation of the sets of integral-treatment perturbed doses was performed by scripting in RayStation, calculating perturbed doses considering fraction-wise random setup errors and systematic range errors, and accumulating the dose considering the anatomy of the weekly cCTs.

Statistical Analysis

Wilcoxon signed-rank tests were performed in SPSS (IBM Corporation, Armonk, NY) to evaluate differences in dose parameters between the plan approaches over the whole patient cohort, and to test differences between nominal dose D_{Nom}, total cumulative doses D_{Cum} and perturbed doses D_{Per0} and D_{PerR}. The differences were considered to be statistically significant with a p-value < 0.05.

6.3 Results

6.3.1 Evaluation of Nominal Plan Doses

For all 20 patients, clinically acceptable treatment plans were generated for the three approaches (PTVb, cRO and aRO). Dose distributions for one patient example are shown in Figure 6.2. The nominal plans D_{Nom} fulfilled the clinical specification of 95% of the prescribed dose levels delivered to the 98% of both target volumes ($D_{98\%} \geq 95\%$) in all cases.

The $D_{98\%}$ doses were smaller for both robustly optimized plans, with a median value over the whole patient cohort for low- and high-risk CTV of 98.2% and 97.9% for cRO, and 97.5% and 97.4% for aRO, respectively, compared to the PTVb plan with median $D_{98\%}$ values of

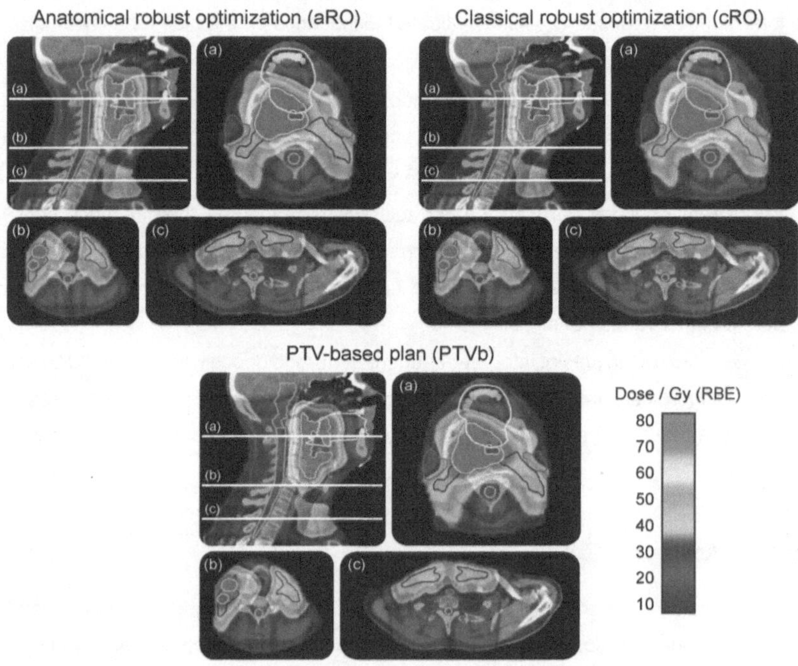

Figure 6.2. Dose distributions for PTVb, cRO and aRO plans for an exemplary patient. White lines in the sagittal view indicate the transversal slice position. Low-risk CTV is delineated in dark brown, whereas high-risk CTV is delineated in pink. The delineated OARs are the same as in Figure 5.1.

99.3% and 98.7%, respectively. In the high-risk region, no volumes $> 2\%$ exceeded 107% of the prescribed dose for all plans.

The clinical objectives for the OARs spinal cord, brainstem and contralateral parotid gland were fulfilled in all cases. For the other OARs, in some cases the doses were higher than the clinical objective, since an important portion of the organ was inside the CTV. Thus, no additional dose sparing was achievable without compromising the CTV coverage. Significant higher D_{mean} doses to the ipsilateral parotid gland, larynx and pharyngeal constrictor muscles were delivered by the PTVb approach, compared with both robustly optimized plans ($p < 0.001$). Moreover, slight but significant higher D_{mean} doses to oral mucosa and esophageal inlet muscle were found for the aRO approach, compared to the cRO plan ($p < 0.028$).

Integral doses to the normal tissue were calculated on the planning CT following the method described by Yang et al. (2009): first, the normal tissue was defined as the entire volume of all CT slices where the CTVs were contoured, plus additional 2 cm superior and inferior, minus the CTV contours. The integral dose to the normal tissue is defined as its volume times its mean dose, measured in Gy·L. The integral dose to the normal tissue was significantly higher for the PTVb and aRO plans in comparison to the cRO plan ($p < 0.001$), with median (range) values over the entire patient cohort of 111.9 Gy·L (70.3–143.3 Gy), 112.9 Gy·L (69.2–146.9 Gy) and 104.8 Gy·L (66.8–134.1 Gy), respectively. Detailed tabulated data can be found in the Appendix, Tables B.2 and B.4.

6.3.2 Evaluation of Plan Robustness Against Uncertainties

Evaluation of Weekly and Total Cumulative Doses

The target coverage during the treatment course showed a degradation on the first week for the PTVb plan in three cases, with minimum $D_{98\%}$ values of 88.9% and 89.8% for low- and high-risk CTV, respectively. Regarding the robust optimized plans, one case showed a decrease in target coverage in the cRO plan, with $D_{98\%}$ values of 93.8% and 94.8% for low- and high-risk CTV, respectively. The aRO approach was able to keep the target coverage above 95%.

In the following weeks additional patients showed target coverage degradation in the case of PTVb plans. Median $D_{98\%}$ doses averaged over the whole patient cohort decreased to values down to 4.4 percentage points during the treatment course, in comparison to the

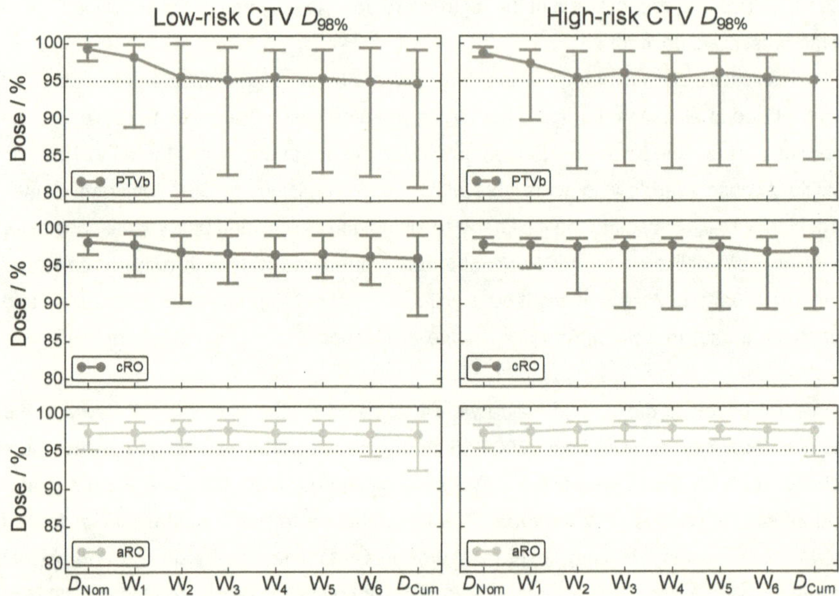

Figure 6.3. Graphical representation of CTV target coverage over time for the whole patient cohort comparing the three plans. Nominal dose (D_{Nom}), weekly cumulative doses of week 1–6 (W_n) and total cumulative doses (D_{Cum}) are depicted. The central dot represents the median value over the patient cohort, the lower and upper error bar represent the minimum and maximum value over the patient cohort, respectively. The dotted line represents the clinical objective ($D_{98\%} \geq 95\%$).

nominal dose. The same was observed for cRO plans, whereas aRO plans could preserve the target coverage without higher variations, until the sixth week, where one case showed a degradation of the low-risk CTV $D_{98\%}$ dose to 94.3%. A visual representation of the weekly cumulative $D_{98\%}$ values for the whole patient cohort is depicted in Figure 6.3. Detailed tabulated data can be found in the Appendix, Table B.1.

The total cumulative doses D_{Cum}, which represent the simulated dose delivered to the patient considering variations in the anatomy during the treatment course, revealed a degradation of the target coverage below 95% for the PTVb plan in 10 out of 20 patients. The median (minimum) $D_{98\%}$ values for these 10 cases were 90.3% (80.8%) and 89.9% (84.5%) for low- and high-risk CTV, respectively. This finding illustrates and confirms that a simple margin expansion from the CTV to the PTV alone cannot account for anatomical variations

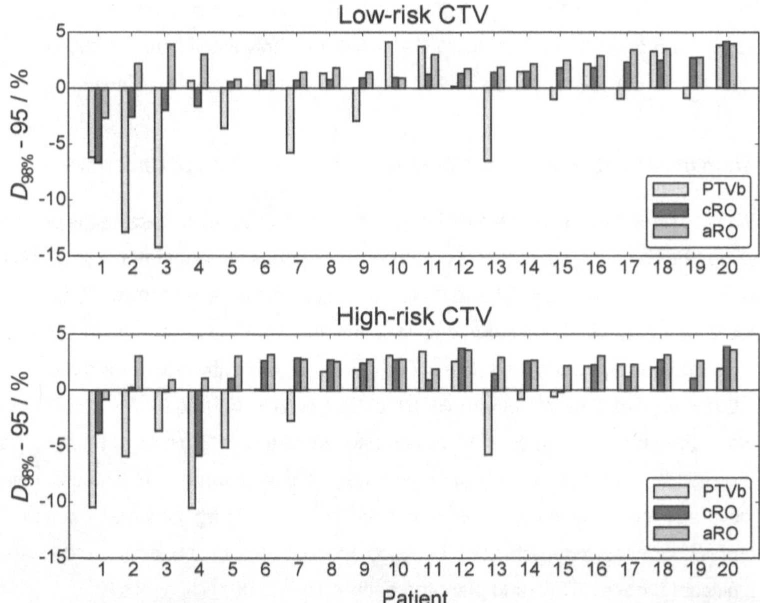

Figure 6.4. Difference between $D_{98\%}$ and objective value (95%) for the total cumulative dose calculated for each patient: a negative value means target coverage below the clinical objective.

during the treatment course, being in line with previous studies. Although the CTV coverage maintained clinically acceptable in ten patients, a plan adaptation would be needed in the remaining 10 patients.

Likewise, the cRO approach was not sufficient to account for positioning and treatment-induced anatomical variation in some cases. Five out of 20 patients showed target coverage degradation, with total cumulative median (minimum) $D_{98\%}$ values across the 5 cases of 93.4% (88.4%) in low-risk CTV and 94.4% (89.2%) in high-risk CTV. These patients would undergo plan adaptation following the intervention criterion. Conversely, the aRO approach was able to preserve the target coverage in acceptable clinical levels in all except for one patient, where the $D_{98\%}$ values were reduced to 92.4% and 94.2% for low- and high-risk CTV, respectively. Figure 6.4 shows the difference between the total cumulative dose with the clinical objective of 95% per patient. Slight but significant higher D_{mean} values compared to the nominal dose were found in spinal cord (cRO: $p < 0.001$; aRO: $p = 0.005$), ipsilateral parotid gland (cRO: $p = 0.008$; aRO: $p = 0.01$) and constrictor muscles (aRO: $p = 0.008$). The dose to the remaining OARs did not show significant variations between D_{Nom} and D_{Cum}. Detailed tabulated data can be found in the Appendix, Tables B.2 and B.4.

Evaluation of Robustness Against Additional Setup and Range Uncertainties

The plan robustness was evaluated for both, cRO and aRO plans, extracting the worst-case values from the calculated cumulative perturbed doses considering anatomy variations plus fraction-wise setup errors (D_{Per0}) and additionally systematic range errors (D_{PerR}).

Considering anatomical and setup uncertainties, the worst-case $D_{98\%}$ values calculated from the 10 cumulative perturbed doses D_{Per0} were significantly worse for the cRO plans ($p < 0.001$), with median (minimum) values of 95.6% (87.2%) and 96.3% (88.7%) for the low- and high-risk CTV, respectively, in comparison to the aRO plans with $D_{98\%}$ values of 96.6% (91.5%) and 97.5% (93.9%) respectively. This is in agreement with the observed target coverage reduction in D_{Cum}. Moreover, the reduction in target coverage due to the inclusion of random setup uncertainties D_{Per0} compared to the total cumulative doses D_{Cum} was significant for both CTVs and plan approaches ($p \leq 0.001$).

Considering additional range uncertainties, the worst-case $D_{98\%}$ values from 20 perturbed doses D_{PerR} showed the same trend, with median (minimum) values for the cRO approach of 95.2% (86.1%) and 96% (87.2%) for low- and high-risk CTV, respectively,

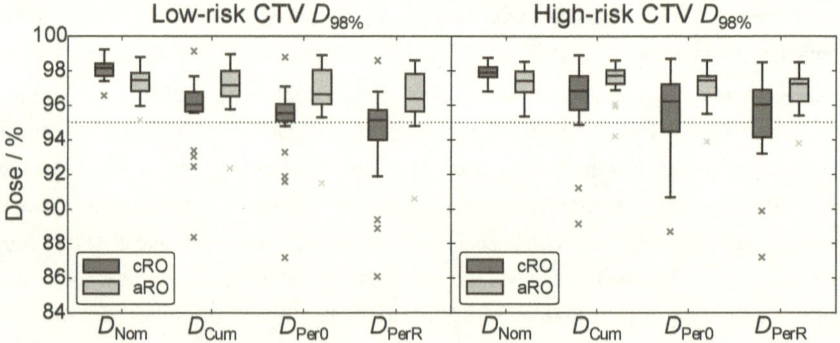

Figure 6.5. Comparison of target coverage ($D_{98\%}$) with cRO (blue) and aRO (orange) plans in nominal dose (D_{Nom}), total cumulative dose (D_{Cum}) and worst-case of the 10 perturbed doses considering setup errors (D_{Per0}) and of the 20 perturbed doses considering range errors (D_{PerR}) for all patients.

Table 6.3. Step-wise target coverage degradation due to the influence of anatomy variation (D_{Cum}), setup errors (D_{Per0}) and range errors (D_{PerR}), in percentage points for the whole patient cohort, median (range).

		cRO	aRO
Low-risk CTV $D_{98\%}$			
	$D_{\mathrm{Nom}}-D_{\mathrm{Cum}}$	1.8 (0.1–9.2)	-0.2 (-0.7–4.2)
	$D_{\mathrm{Cum}}-D_{\mathrm{Per0}}$	0.5 (0.0–1.9)	0.2 (-0.2–1.0)
	$D_{\mathrm{Per0}}-D_{\mathrm{PerR}}$	0.6 (0.1–2.8)	0.4 (-0.1–0.9)
	$D_{\mathrm{Nom}}-D_{\mathrm{PerR}}$	2.9 (0.6–11.5)	0.6 (-0.4–6.0)
High-risk CTV $D_{98\%}$			
	$D_{\mathrm{Nom}}-D_{\mathrm{Cum}}$	1.1 (-0.3–7.9)	-0.3 (-1.9–2.1)
	$D_{\mathrm{Cum}}-D_{\mathrm{Per0}}$	0.5 (0.0–2.1)	0.3 (0.0–2.4)
	$D_{\mathrm{Per0}}-D_{\mathrm{PerR}}$	0.3 (0.0–1.5)	0.2 (-0.1–0.7)
	$D_{\mathrm{Nom}}-D_{\mathrm{PerR}}$	1.7 (-0.1–9.9)	0.1 (-1.6–2.5)

Abbreviations: cRO, classical robustly optimized plan; aRO, anatomical robustly optimized plan; CTV, clinical target volume; $D_{98\%}$, dose to the 98% of the volume.

compared to 96.4% (90.6%) and 97.2% (93.8%) for the aRO plans, respectively. The differences between D_{Per0} and D_{PerR} were not large but statistically significant ($p < 0.001$), with median differences of 0.6 pp and 0.3 pp for low- and high risk CTV in cRO plans, and 0.3 pp and 0.2 pp in aRO plans, respectively (Table 6.3). A general overview of the CTV coverage for the entire patient cohort considering the different uncertainties is depicted in Figure 6.5.

The variation of target coverage ($D_{98\%}$) per patient between the overall investigated cumulative perturbed doses, i.e. the total parameter width, was in general larger for cRO plans, indicating a reduced plan robustness for the cRO cases, with median (maximum) values from the 20 patients of 1.5 (5.5) and 1.0 (3.9) for low- and high-risk CTV, respectively, in comparison to aRO, with values of 1.0 (2.9) and 0.6 (3.3), respectively, as shown in Figure 6.6, and tabulated in the Appendix, Table B.3.

The number of cumulative perturbed doses where the coverage of both target volumes was sufficient was of mean ± standard deviation (percentage) of 20.4 ± 12.4 (68.0%) for the cRO plan, compared to 28.2 ± 6.8 (93.8%) for the aRO plan. For each CTV, the number of perturbed scenarios fulfilling the clinical target coverage objective was 22.3 ± 12.0 (74.2%) and 22.5 ± 12.0 (74.8%) for low- and high-risk CTV, respectively, in comparison

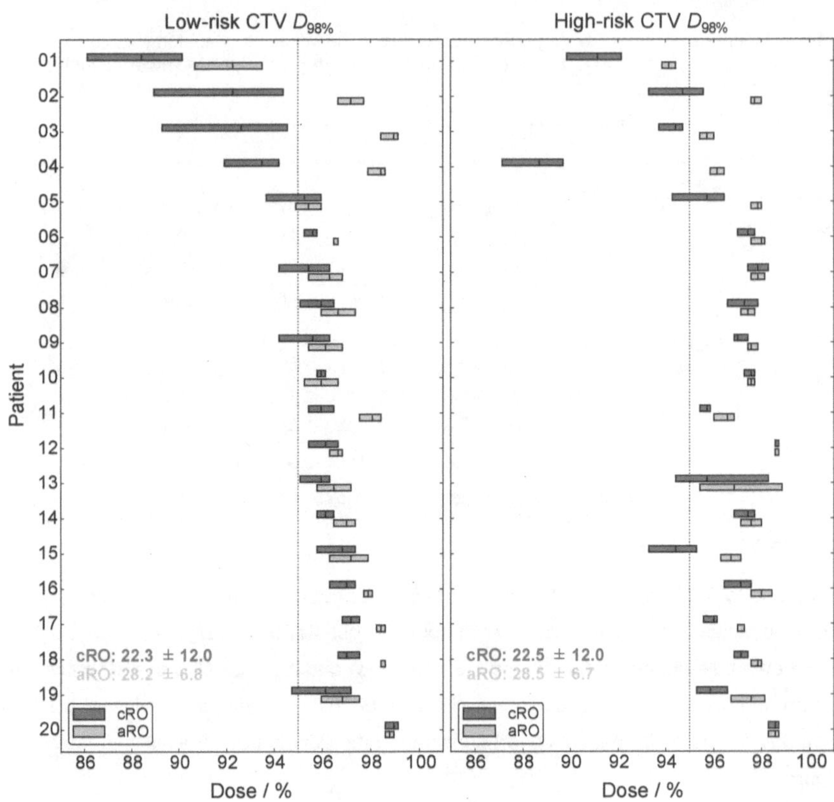

Figure 6.6. CTV $D_{98\%}$ statistics for the set of 30 integral-treatment perturbed doses per bilateral HNSCC plan and patient. The central line in each box represents the median value. The dashed lines represent the clinical objective (95%). The scenarios fulfilling the clinical objective are written for each approach (mean ± standard deviation).

to 28.2 ± 6.8 (93.8%) and 28.5 ± 6.7 (95.0%), respectively, for the aRO plan.

The difference in the OAR dose parameters between D_{Cum}, D_{Per0} and D_{PerR} per plan were small but significant ($p \leq 0.002$ for all OARs). The doses to the spinal cord and brainstem remained below the objectives in all cases, as well as the dose to the contralateral parotid gland on the aRO plan. In only one patient the mean dose to the contralateral parotid gland on the cRO plan was above the objective (D_{Per0}: 26.5 Gy; D_{PerR}: 26.9 Gy). Comparing between both plans, slightly higher but significant D_{mean} values were found for the aRO

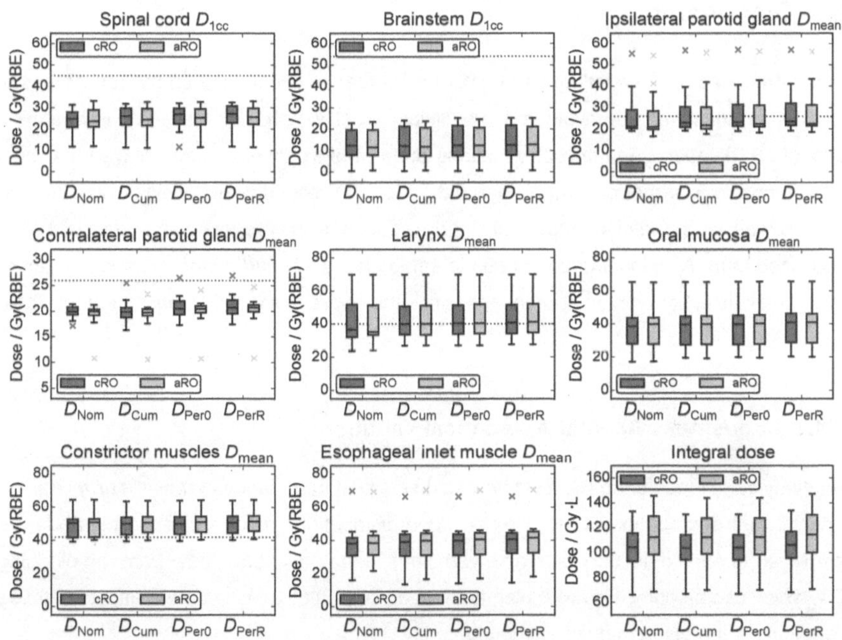

Figure 6.7. Comparison of OAR dose parameters and integral dose to the healthy tissue for cRO (blue) and aRO (orange) plans in nominal dose (D_{Nom}), total cumulative dose (D_{Cum}) and worst-case of the 10 perturbed doses considering setup errors (D_{PerO}) and of the 20 perturbed doses considering range errors (D_{PerR}) for all patients.

plans in oral mucosa, constrictor muscles and esophageal inlet muscle in D_{Cum}, D_{PerO} and D_{PerR} ($p \leq 0.007$, respectively). The results for OARs doses for the overall patient cohort are depicted in Figure 6.7.

The integral dose to the normal tissue was in all cases higher for the aRO plans, being in agreement with what was observed in the nominal doses. For both plans, D_{PerR} values for integral dose showed an increase of the median values by about 1.8 Gy·L compared to the nominal value D_{Nom}, whereas anatomical variation D_{Cum} and setup errors D_{PerO} had no significant differences on the integral dose values compared to D_{Nom}. The results for integral dose for the overall patient cohort are depicted in Figure 6.7. A complete tabulated summary of the evaluated dose parameters for both CTV and OARs can be found in the Appendix, Table B.4.

6.4 Discussion

In the present study, the influence of different sources of uncertainty on the robustness of HNSCC proton plans was evaluated in a clinically realistic scenario based on in-treatment control CT datasets. Anatomical variations during the treatment course played the most important role in target coverage degradation for PTV-based and classical robustly optimized plans, while their influence was clearly reduced by the proposed anatomical robustly optimized plan. Additional uncertainties in setup and range had minor influence on target coverage loss in both robust approaches, since they were optimized against them (cf. Table 6.3).

6.4.1 Robustness Against Anatomical Variations

Anatomy variations during the treatment course are of importance in radiotherapy, leading to important degradation of the planned dose distribution. Image guidance methods are employed to early detect considerable variations in the patient anatomy from the planning CT, which can be combined with plan adaptation strategies to mitigate the effects of these variations in the planned dose distributions.

Patients with bilateral HNSCC irradiation show frequently anatomy variations during the treatment course, e.g. tumor shrinkage and weight loss, which might lead to a degradation in the target coverage and/or a higher dose to the OARs, requiring plan adaptation, especially in proton therapy cases (Barker et al., 2004; Góra et al., 2015; Müller et al., 2015; Thomson et al., 2015; Stützer et al., 2017a). Plan adaptation strategies are usually time consuming, requiring many resources from clinicians, medical physicists and radiation technicians: a new planning CT acquisition, together with volume contouring, treatment replanning and patient-specific quality assurance, which must be executed quickly since the patient is already in treatment and the new adapted plan should be applied as soon as possible. If a treatment planning approach could somehow reduce the need of plan adaptation, there will be a direct benefit and efficacy in the clinical workflow.

In this work, it was shown and confirmed that a simple CTV-to-PTV margin expansion is not sufficient to account for anatomy variations in IMPT HNSCC plans, which is in agreement with previous studies (Barker et al., 2004; Kraan et al., 2013; Brouwer et al., 2015; Góra et al., 2015; Müller et al., 2015; Thomson et al., 2015; Stützer et al., 2017a). Furthermore, a classical robustly optimized plan (cRO) considering uncertainties in patient setup and proton range in the optimization, might also not be sufficient, although it showed a better performance in comparison to the PTV-based plan.

A new robust planning approach was proposed, anatomical robust optimization (aRO), which considers not only setup and range uncertainties in the plan optimization, but also variations in patient positioning, with the inclusion of additional CT datasets in the plan optimization. The aRO plan was able to compensate for variations in anatomy during treatment, preserving the target coverage above clinically acceptable levels during the whole treatment course, with small variations on the OAR dose between cRO and aRO plans. Only integral doses to the healthy tissue were significantly higher for the aRO plans by about 8 Gy·L compared to the cRO approach, although this increase on the integral dose was in general not reflected in the OAR dose parameters, showing only for the oral mucosa and esophageal inlet muscle a slight but significant higher mean dose on the nominal plan. Thus, the price of improved plan robustness against treatment-induced anatomical variations for the aRO plan can be considered as low.

Since the available patient datasets consisted of only one pretreatment planning CT and weekly cCTs acquired during the treatment course, the first two cCT, usually obtained in the first two weeks of treatment, were used for the calculation of aRO plans, with the assumption that the datasets would have been acquired prior treatment as additional planning CTs. In the studied patient cohort, the changes observed in the first two cCT were random patient positioning variations, such as shoulder positioning variation or small rotations in

Table 6.4. Difference (Δ) of the CTV volumes between planning and first, second and last cCTs; median (range) for the cohort of 20 patients. A negative number represents a reduction of the CTV volume on the correspondent cCT and vice-versa. A large median volume reduction can be seen on the last cCT, compared to the first two cCTs.

Clinical target volume	Control CT	Δ Volume (cm^3)
Low-risk CTV	First cCT	6.2 (-35.6–84.3)
	Second cCT	-1.1 (-53.2–89.4)
	Last cCT	-11.8 (-113.5–28.1)
High-risk CTV	First cCT	0.5 (-25.0–65.0)
	Second cCT	-5.0 (-44.7–69.5)
	Last cCT	-16.0 (-83.3–36.7)

Abbreviations: CTV, clinical target volume; cCT, control CT.

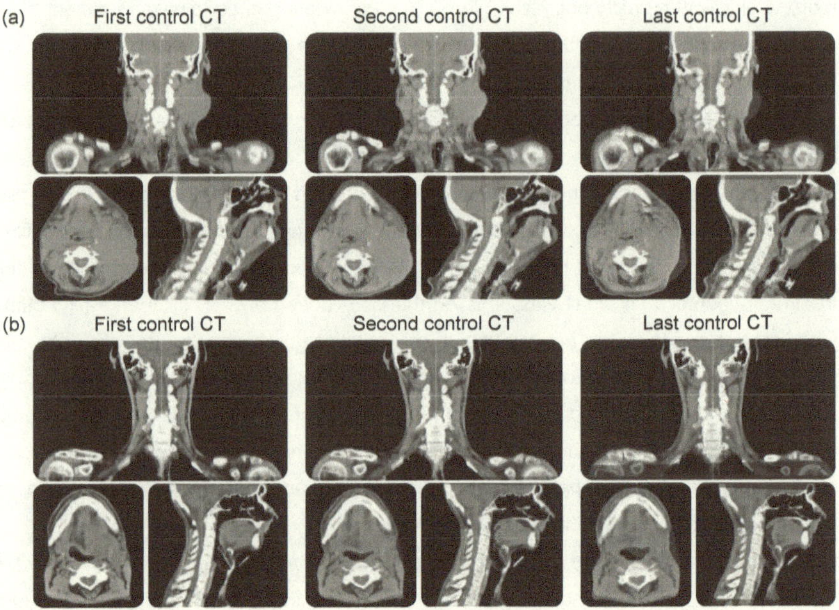

Figure 6.8. Registration of the planning CT (blue) with the correspondent weekly cCT (orange) of two exemplary patients. The patient in (a) shows clearly on the last cCT tumor shrinkage on the left side, whereas the patient in (b) does not show large anatomical variations. Both patients show in the first and second cCT variations of random nature.

the mandible and neck area, as pictured for two patient examples in Figure 6.8. It has been shown that treatment-induced anatomical variations are significant in the last weeks of treatment (Barker et al., 2004; Thomson et al., 2015). Moreover, the variations in the CTV volume in the first two cCT were higher in the last cCT, compared to the first two weekly cCTs used on the plan optimization (Table 6.4).

In principle, the aRO approach is feasible to be implemented into the clinical workflow, by the acquisition of additional pretreatment planing CT datasets. To consider variations in patient positioning, each additional planning CT should be acquired after a complete patient repositioning, in order to image realistic differences in patient positioning as variations of head tilt and rotation, shoulder position, neck flexion, mandible and palate position in HNSCC patients. Further aspects such as the additional patient CT dose and the increased effort in the clinical workflow, should be considered as well. Current advances such as dual-energy CT and iterative reconstruction algorithms, allow for a reduction in the CT dose. Furthermore, new promising approaches, which are able to simulate patient positioning variability by means of biomechanical models, are being investigated (Teske et al., 2017), likewise deep learning methods applied to image datasets (Sahiner et al., 2019).

Further studies have shown that the inclusion of additional anatomy datasets in the planning process can increase the robustness of the plans against anatomical variations. Wang et al. (2017) calculated treatment plans for lung cancer patients using multiple CT optimization, including two CTs in the plan optimization, with the second CT acquired during the treatment course for plan adaptation. The multiple CT plan was compared to a classical robust plan using the single planning CT, and to an additional adaptive robust plan using the second CT. The multiple CT plans showed an increased robustness in comparison to the classical robust plan and the adaptive plan. However, since additional control CT datasets were not available, it remained unclear whether the multiple CT plans were robust against successive anatomical variations.

For sinonasal tumors, van de Water et al. (2018) included synthetic CTs with variable nasal cavity filling in the plan optimization. These plans provided adequate target coverage in a repeated CT acquired during the treatment course in comparison to a PTV-based SFO plan. However, they did not consider additional random anatomical variations outside the manipulated area, and the plan optimization and further evaluation did not include additional uncertainties in setup and range.

In summary, neither PTV-based planning nor classical robust optimization were sufficient to account for anatomical variations during the treatment course. Including additional CT image datasets accounting for variations in patient positioning in the robust plan optimization can improve the robustness of the plans against anatomy variability during the treatment course. In addition, the importance of an early detection of anatomical variations during the treatment course in proton therapy is underlined, making use of in-room image guidance systems and potentially *in vivo* range verification techniques.

6.4.2 Robustness Against Additional Setup and Range Uncertainties

To generate robustly optimized plans, the values for setup and range uncertainty must be defined and included in the optimizer. Van der Voort et al. (2016) determined recipes for the assessment of setup and range error parameters to be used in minimax robustly optimized plans in oropharyngeal cancer patients. For bilateral cases, they determined a range error of 3–4% and a setup error of 3.3–3.4 mm. The values used in this study, 3 mm setup error and 3.5% range error, are smaller for the setup error compared to the recipe. However, they are in good agreement with previously published studies regarding robust optimization for HNSCC cases (Liu et al., 2013a; Liu et al., 2013b; Li et al., 2015b; van Dijk et al., 2016; Stützer et al., 2017b).

The robustness of proton plans against setup and range uncertainties has been evaluated in previous studies to show the advantage of robustly optimized plans against PTV-based plans. In early studies, the worst-case dose distribution introduced by Lomax et al. (2001) was generated from a set of fixed error scenarios and compared to the nominal dose (Liu et al., 2013a; Liu et al., 2013b; Li et al., 2015b). However, one disadvantage of this method is the neglect of the fractionation effect, i.e. counterbalancing the impact of random setup errors between fractions, and therefore overestimating the dose perturbation. Later, methods including the fractionation effect in the robustness analysis have been introduced, considering the convergence of fraction-wise setup errors in the dose distributions (Park et al., 2013; Lowe et al., 2016; Stützer et al., 2017b).

In this study, the fractionation effect was accounted by the generation of fraction-wise random setup errors, simulating a complete fractionated treatment delivery, whereas the range uncertainty was considered as a systematic error. The analyzed worst-case values from the cumulative perturbed dose distributions avoid an overconservative evaluation, since these values might be a real dose delivery after a fractionated treatment. For the evaluation, this study considered as well the anatomical variations during the treatment course. Thus, the calculated perturbed doses, considering three sources of uncertainty, i.e. fraction-wise random setup errors, systematic range errors and weekly anatomy variations, simulate a realistic treatment course.

Since both cRO and aRO plans were optimized to be robust against setup and range uncertainties, they had a minor influence on the target coverage degradation. As mentioned before, anatomical variations played the most critical role regarding CTV coverage degradation (cf. Table 6.3). The plan robustness might be approximated during the treatment course by assessment of cumulative doses with in-treatment acquired control CTs, providing an estimate of the dose degradation due to the influence of variations in the anatomy during the treatment course.

6.4.3 Study Limitations

Patient dataset The image datasets used in this study, i.e. planning and control CTs, were taken from patients who received photon therapy. In the clinical proton therapy practice in Dresden, different immobilization devices, i.e. patient-specific head and neck support and masks, are used. Moreover, it was implicitly assumed that a patient undergoing proton therapy would, when receiving the same prescribed fraction dose and schedule, experience similar anatomical variations during the treatment course as in photon therapy. The anatomical variations covered in the investigated cohort of 20 patients might be limited and it should be considered that more severe treatment-induced anatomical variations might occur in other patients. Prospective studies with HNSCC patients treated with IMPT and the assessment of the degree of anatomical variations with this treatment modality would be beneficial.

Treatment planning approach Since additional pre-treatment planning CTs were not available for the studied patient cohort, the aRO plans were calculated using the planning CT and the first two cCTs in the plan optimization, corresponding usually to the first two weeks of treatment. In three patients, cCT of the third week was used, since the first or second weekly cCT was not available. The cCTs included in the optimization did not present treatment-induced anatomy variations such as tumor shrinkage, but variations in patient positioning, especially in the shoulder and mandible region (Figure 6.8). Therefore, it can be assumed that if additional planning CTs are acquired with complete patient repositioning between scans, the conclusions drawn from this study will hold true.

The same treatment field configuration for each patient was used for the IMPT plans, using a 3-field arrangement as proposed in previous publications (Cozzi et al., 2001; Steneker et al., 2006; Kraan et al., 2013; Quan et al., 2013; Frank et al., 2014; van Dijk et al., 2016). A study by van der Laan et al. (2013) suggested that the OAR sparing can be improved if the treatment field number is increased. However, additional studies by Kraan et al. (2013) and van Dijk et al. (2016) showed no significant changes in the plan robustness with an increased treatment field number. Moreover, other treatment field configurations might improve the OAR sparing and reduce secondary tissue complications, for example mucositis by dose sparing of the oral mucosa (Stützer et al., 2017b).

Image registration uncertainties The deformable image registration (DIR) procedure can lead to uncertainties in contour propagation and in the calculation of cumulative doses. Uncertainties in the image datasets, such as image artifacts, motion and large variations in the anatomy might be a source of error in the registration. Similarly, the rigid registration between planning and control CTs might be not satisfactory, if for instance significant rotations in shoulders and mandible region are present. Therefore, an exact patient positioning method between fractions, checking patient rotations and shoulder position is crucial to ensure an accurate image registration.

Regarding the use of DIR for dose accumulation, regions of higher dose gradients and deficient image contrast can present uncertainties in dose recalculation on the cCT and further dose accumulation on the planning CT. These uncertainties in DIR are a general limitation of planning studies performing dose accumulation (Brock et al., 2017; Paganelli et al., 2018; Ribeiro et al., 2018). Possible errors in the contours propagated from the planning CT to the cCTs were reduced in this study by a revision by the radiation oncologist on each cCT.

Dose statistics evaluation Only CTV coverage degradation was chosen as a trigger for adaptation. However, also OAR constraint violations might be used as additional trigger for replanning, without loss of generality in the presented results.

Perturbed dose calculation For the calculation of integral-treatment perturbed doses, random fraction setup errors were drawn from a Gaussian distribution with mean of 0 mm and standard deviation of 1.5 mm. Since institutional values for setup error in bilateral HNSCC patients were not yet determined, the value of 1.5 mm was chosen following previous studies (van Kranen et al., 2009; Amelio et al., 2013; Ciardo et al., 2015; Lowe et al., 2016; Stützer et al., 2017b).

The calculation to generate treatment-wise perturbed dose distributions was intensively time consuming, being up to 9 hours per plan (for a total of 30 cumulated perturbed doses) per patient within the used version of RayStation. For each cumulative perturbed dose, the algorithm calculates first the 33 perturbed fraction doses with different setup errors, and deforms them onto the planning CT for accumulation.

6.5 Conclusions

Anatomical variations during the treatment course play the most critical role in target coverage degradation of IMPT PTV-based and classical robustly optimized plans for HNSCC. The proposed anatomical robustly optimized approach preserves the target coverage due to anatomy variations in most of the cases, maintaining similar robustness against setup and range uncertainties as the cRO plans, without increasing the dose to the OARs.

The clinical implementation of aRO is in principle feasible, acquiring additional planning CT datasets for the plan optimization. Additional dosimetric and organizational aspects must be weighted against the expected benefit in improved plan robustness and in the clinical wokflow by a reduced need of replanning. In addition, the importance of image guidance in proton therapy is underlined, to allow for dose recalculation and by that enabling an early detection of target coverage loss.

7

Summary

Intensity modulated proton therapy (IMPT) in head and neck squamous cell carcinoma (HNSCC) offers superior advantages over conventional photon therapy, by generating high conformal doses to the target volume and improved sparing of the organ at risks (OARs). Besides, robust treatment planning approaches, which account for uncertainties directly into the plan optimization process, are able to generate high quality plans robust against uncertainties compared to a PTV margin expansion approach.

During radiation treatment, patients are prone to present anatomical variations during the treatment course, which can be random deviations in patient positioning, as well as treatment-induced tumor shrinkage and patient weight variations. For IMPT plans using a PTV margin expansion, these anatomical variations might disturb the calculated nominal plan, with a decrease to the dose delivered to the target volume and/or increased dose to the OARs above its tolerance, and a plan adaptation might be needed. However, the influence of these anatomical variations in robustly optimized plans for HNSCC entities has not been determined.

The first part of this book compared two proton therapy methods, single-field optimiza-tion (SFO) and multi-field optimization (MFO), applied to the treatment of unilateral HNSCC target volumes, consisting of a cohort of 8 patients. For each method, a PTV-based and a robustly optimized plan were generated, resulting in four plans per patient. The four plans showed adequate target coverage on the nominal plan, with larger doses to the ipsilateral parotid gland for both SFO approaches. No plan showed a clear advantage when variations in the anatomy during the treatment course were considered, and the same was observed considering additional setup and range uncertainties. Hence, no plan showed a decisive superiority regarding plan robustness and potential need of replanning.

In the second part of this book, an anatomical robustly optimized plan approach was proposed (aRO), which considers additional CT datasets in the plan optimization, representing random non-rigid patient positioning variations. The aRO approach was compared to a classical robustly optimized plan (cRO) and a PTV-based approach for a cohort of 20 bilateral HNSCC patients. PTV-based and cRO approaches were not sufficient to account for weekly anatomical variations, showing a degradation in the target coverage in 10 and 5 of 20 cases, respectively. Conversely, the proposed aRO approach was able to preserve the target coverage in 19 of 20 cases, with only one patient requiring plan adaptation. An extended robustness analysis conducted on both cRO and aRO plan approaches considering weekly anatomical variations, setup and range errors, showed that the variations in anatomy were the most critical variable for loss in target coverage, while setup and range uncertainties played a minor role. The price of the increased plan robustness for the aRO approach was a significant larger integral dose to the healthy tissue, compared to the cRO plan. However, the increase in integral dose was not reflected on the planned dose to the OARs, which were comparable between both plans. Therefore, the price for a superior plan robustness can be considered as low.

In the current clinical practice, the implementation of the aRO approach would be able to reduce the need of plan adaptation. For its application, the acquisition of additional planning CT datasets, considering a complete patient repositioning between scans is required, in order to simulate random non-rigid position variations as simulated in this study by the use of the first two weekly cCTs in the plan optimization. Further studies using multiple planning CT acquisition, including strategies to reduce the patient CT dose such as dual-energy CT and iterative reconstruction algorithms, are needed to confirm the presented findings. Additionally, the aRO approach applied to other body sites and entities might also be investigated. In near future, further in-room imaging methods such as cone-beam CT and magnetic resonance imaging, optimized for proton therapy, might be used to acquire additional datasets. Moreover, alternative approaches capable of modeling variations in patient positioning as biomechanical models and deep learning methods might be able to generate *in silico* additional image datasets for use in proton treatment planning.

In summary, this book proposes an additional contribution for robust treatment planning in IMPT, with the generation of treatment plans robust against anatomy variations, together with setup and range uncertainties, which can benefit the clinical workflow by reducing the need of plan adaptation.

8

Zusammenfassung

Intensitätsmodulierte Protonentherapie (IMPT) beim Plattenepithelkarzinom des Kopf-Hals-Bereiches ist der konventionellen Photonentherapie weit überlegen, durch eine hohe Konformität der Dosis auf das Zielvolumen und geringe Belastung der Risikoorgane. Darüber hinaus können robuste Bestrahlungsplanungsansätze, die Unsicherheiten direkt in den Planoptimierungsprozess einbeziehen, im Vergleich zu einem PTV-basierten Plan hochwertige Pläne generieren.

Während des Behandlungsverlaufs zeigen Patienten anatomische Veränderungen, wie zufällige Abweichungen bei der Patientenpositionierung sowie behandlungsbedingte Tumorschrumpfung und Patientgewichtsabweichungen. Bei PTV-basierten IMPT Plänen können diese anatomischen Variationen den berechneten Nominalplan stören, mit in der Folge einer Verringerung der Dosis im Zielvolumen und/oder einer erhöhten Dosis an den Risikoorganen über ihre Toleranz. Dadurch wird eine Anpassung des Bestrahlungsplans erforderlich. Der Einfluss dieser anatomischen Veränderung auf robust optimierte Pläne wurde jedoch noch nicht untersucht.

Der erste Teil der vorliegenden Arbeit verglich Protonentherapiemethoden, die Single-Field-Optimierung (SFO) und die Multi-Field-Optimierung (MFO), die auf die Behandlung 8 Kopf-Hals Patienten angewendet wurden, deren Hals einseitig bestrahlt wurde. Für jede Methode wurden ein PTV-basierter und ein robust optimierter Plan erstellt, insgesamt vier Pläne pro Patient. Die vier Pläne zeigten eine angemessene Erfassung des Zielvolumens, mit höherer Dosis der ipsilateralen Parotis in beiden SFO Ansätze. Kein Plan zeigte einen klaren Vorteil, wenn Variationen in der Anatomie während des Behandlungsverlaufs, und zusätzliche Setup- und Reichweiteunsicherheiten berücksichtigt wurden. Daher wies kein Plan eine entscheidende Überlegenheit hinsichtlich der Planrobustheit und des potenziellen Nachplanungsbedarfs auf.

Im zweiten Teil der vorliegenden Arbeit wurde ein anatomisch robuster Optimierungsansatz (aRO) vorgeschlagen, der zuzätzliche CT-Datensätze in der Planoptimierung berücksichtigt, die zufällige Variationen der Patientenpositionierung darstellen. Der aRO Ansatz wurde für eine Kohorte von 20 bilateralen Kopf-Hals-Tumoren Patienten mit einem klassischen robusten Optimierungsansatz (cRO) und einem PTV-basierten Ansatz verglichen. PTV-basierte und cRO Ansätze reichten nicht aus, um wöchentliche anatomische Veränderungen zu berücksichtigen. In 10 bzw. 5 von 20 Fälle zeigten sie eine Verschlechterung der Erfassung des Zielvolumens. Der vorgeschlagene aRO Ansatz behielt die Erfassung des Zielvolumens in 19 von 20 Fällen bei, wobei nur ein Patient eine Plananpassung benötigte. Eine erweiterte Robustheitsanalyse, die wöchentlichen anatomischen Veränderungen, Setup- und Reichweitefehler berücksichtigt, wurde für cRO und aRO Planungsansätze durchgeführt. Die Variationen in der Anatomie waren die kritischste Variable für den Verlust der Zielvolumendosis, während Setup- und Reichweiteunsicherheiten eine untergeordnete Rolle spielten. Der Preis für die erhöhte Planrobustheit für den aRO Ansatz war eine signifikant größere integrale Dosis für das gesunde Gewebe, im Vergleich zum cRO Plan. Die Erhöhung der integralen Dosis spiegelte sich jedoch nicht in der geplanten Dosis für die Risikoorgane wider, die zwischen beiden Plänen vergleichbar war. Daher kann der Preis für eine überlegene Planrobustheit als niedrig angesehen werden.

In der gegenwärtigen klinischen Praxis könnte durch die Implementierung des aRO Ansatzes die Notwendigkeit einer Plananpassung verringert werden. Für seine Anwendung ist die Erfassung zusätzlicher CT-Planungsdatensätze erforderlich, bei denen eine vollständige Neupositionierung des Patienten zwischen den Scans berücksichtigt wird, um zufällige Positionsschwankungen zu simulieren, wie sie in dieser Studie unter Verwendung der ersten beiden wöchentlichen Kontroll-CTs in der Planoptimierung simuliert wurden. Weitere Studien unter Verwendung mit mehreren CT-Planungsdatensätzen sind erforderlich, um die präsentierten Ergebnisse zu bestätigen. Strategien zur Reduzierung der Patientendosis wie Dual-Energy-CT und iterative Rekonstruktionsalgorithmen können in Betracht gezogen werden. Darüber hinaus könnte der aRO Ansatz auf andere Körperstellen untersucht werden. In naher Zukunft könnten weitere bildgebende Verfahren, wie Cone-Beam-CT und Magnetresonanztomographie, die für die Protonentherapie optimiert sind, verwendet werden, um zusätzliche Datensätze zu erwerben. Darüber hinaus könnten alternative Ansätze zur Modellierung von Variationen bei der Patientenpositionierung als biomechanische Modelle und Deep-Learning-Methode zusätzliche *in silico* CT-Datensätze für die Protonentherapie generieren.

Zusammenfassend trägt diese Arbeit zur robusten Bestrahlungsplanung in der IMPT bei: sie präsentiert den Ansatz, robuste Bestrahlungspläne unter zusätzlicher Einbeziehung anatomischer Veränderung zu erstellen. Mit diesem neuen Ansatz kann der klinische Arbeitsablauf durch die Reduzierung des Bedarfs an Plananpassungen verbessert werden.

Appendix

The next sections present supplementary material for both unilateral and bilateral HNSCC studies. The data are tabulated here to improve the readability of the book main chapters.

A Supplementary Material for the Unilateral HNSCC Study

Table A.1. Total width of the CTV $D_{98\%}$ parameter from the set of unilateral HNSCC integral-treatment perturbed doses D_{PerNom} and D_{PerCum}; median (range) for the cohort of 8 patients.

ROI and Metric	Plan	D_{PerNom}		D_{PerCum}	
Low-risk CTV	MFO_{PTV}	1.8	(1.1–9.3)	1.9	(0.8–9.7)
$D_{98\%}$ (%)	MFO_{Rob}	0.8	(0.5–1.2)	0.9	(0.2–2.0)
	SFO_{PTV}	0.6	(0.4–1.5)	0.7	(0.4–2.4)
	SFO_{Rob}	0.5	(0.3–1.3)	0.6	(0.3–2.9)
High-risk CTV	MFO_{PTV}	1.8	(0.8–3.0)	1.4	(0.6–5.9)
$D_{98\%}$ (%)	MFO_{Rob}	0.9	(0.6–1.2)	1.5	(0.6–2.1)
	SFO_{PTV}	0.6	(0.3–1.4)	0.7	(0.4–3.8)
	SFO_{Rob}	0.9	(0.5–4.1)	1.2	(0.7–3.0)

Abbreviations: ROI, region of interest; CTV, clinical target volume; $D_{98\%}$, dose to the 98% of the volume.

Table A.2. Dose statistics for the four unilateral HNSCC plan approaches; median (range) for the cohort of 8 patients. The perturbed doses correspond to the worst-case values considering the anatomy of the planning CT (D_{PerNom}) and the anatomy of the control CTs (D_{PerCum})

ROI and Metric	Plan	Nominal dose D_{Nom}		Cumulative dose D_{Cum}		Perturbed dose D_{PerNom}		Perturbed dose D_{PerCum}	
Low-risk CTV	MFO_{PTV}	99.5	(99.2–99.8)	99.6	(95.8–100.2)	98.7	(90.3–99.3)	98.2	(89.8–99.6)
$D_{98\%}$ (%)	MFO_{Rob}	97.5	(96.9–98.8)	97.8	(96.9–98.5)	98.3	(97.5–98.8)	98.1	(94.8–98.9)
	SFO_{PTV}	100.0	(98.0–100.5)	100.0	(95.5–100.7)	100.0	(97.5–100.7)	99.6	(94.1–100.5)
	SFO_{Rob}	98.5	(97.0–100.4)	98.7	(95.6–100.4)	99.1	(96.9–100.8)	98.8	(93.6–100.5)
$D_{2\%}$ (%)	MFO_{PTV}	117.5	(113.5–122.8)	118.4	(113.0–124.2)	119.9	(115.7–124.2)	120.4	(113.3–125.1)
	MFO_{Rob}	106.0	(105.1–108.0)	106.4	(104.9–108.7)	106.4	(106.0–108.3)	107.1	(106.1–110.0)
	SFO_{PTV}	118.8	(115.5–123.6)	119.1	(115.0–123.7)	120.0	(116.7–123.8)	120.5	(115.7–125.3)
	SFO_{Rob}	108.6	(107.4–111.2)	108.9	(106.3–112.2)	109.7	(108.6–113.3)	110.6	(107.8–113.8)
High-risk CTV	MFO_{PTV}	99.4	(99.0–99.6)	99.6	(97.9–101.4)	98.0	(97.2–99.1)	98.6	(93.0–100.9)
$D_{98\%}$ (%)	MFO_{Rob}	98.5	(97.4–99.8)	98.0	(94.8–98.7)	97.7	(96.1–98.7)	96.3	(93.4–96.8)
	SFO_{PTV}	99.8	(99.5–100.8)	99.8	(97.0–100.6)	99.8	(98.5–100.4)	99.5	(94.0–100.0)
	SFO_{Rob}	99.3	(98.3–100.6)	98.2	(96.9–99.9)	98.0	(94.2–99.5)	96.6	(95.1–98.4)
$D_{2\%}$ (%)	MFO_{PTV}	104.5	(104.1–105.1)	105.0	(104.3–109.6)	105.1	(103.9–105.7)	106.0	(104.4–112.0)
	MFO_{Rob}	105.6	(104.6–106.3)	103.3	(104.3–105.5)	104.8	(103.7–105.2)	104.7	(104.1–105.5)
	SFO_{PTV}	104.4	(103.6–104.6)	103.9	(103.2–104.3)	104.0	(103.3–104.1)	103.5	(103.0–104.3)
	SFO_{Rob}	105.0	(104.5–105.7)	104.5	(103.8–105.0)	104.4	(103.9–104.8)	103.9	(103.4–104.5)
Spinal cord	MFO_{PTV}	1.8	(0.5–10.0)	2.0	(1.4–10.8)	3.3	(0.8–11.2)	3.8	(2.0–12.4)
D_{1cc} (Gy)	MFO_{Rob}	2.0	(0.6–7.5)	2.3	(1.3–8.5)	3.3	(0.9–9.2)	3.6	(2.1–10.4)
	SFO_{PTV}	1.8	(0.4–12.1)	2.0	(1.0–13.0)	3.0	(0.8–13.9)	3.3	(1.6–14.9)
	SFO_{Rob}	1.7	(0.5–9.8)	2.2	(1.3–11.0)	3.0	(0.9–11.9)	3.3	(2.2–13.0))

(Continued on next page)

Table A.2. (Continued)

ROI and Metric	Plan	Nominal dose D_{Nom}	Cumulative dose D_{Cum}	Perturbed dose D_{PerNom}	Perturbed dose D_{PerCum}
Brainstem	MFO_{PTV}	3.3 (0.1–5.3)	3.9 (0.0–5.6)	5.2 (0.2–7.5)	6.4 (0.1–9.4)
D_{1cc} (Gy)	MFO_{Rob}	3.1 (0.0–4.6)	3.4 (0.0–6.4)	4.1 (0.1–6.6)	5.2 (0.1–8.0)
	SFO_{PTV}	3.6 (0.0–6.2)	4.0 (0.0–6.4)	5.7 (0.0–8.4)	6.3 (0.0–9.3)
	SFO_{Rob}	3.1 (0.0–5.1)	3.6 (0.0–6.5)	4.8 (0.0–7.6)	5.6 (0.0–8.4)
Ipsilateral parotid gland	MFO_{PTV}	25.5 (24.0–29.8)	27.9 (24.1–31.5)	27.6 (26.2–31.6)	29.6 (26.1–33.4)
D_{median} (Gy)	MFO_{Rob}	24.8 (23.4–27.2)	25.1 (23.1–28.8)	26.9 (25.9–29.3)	26.9 (25.4–30.8)
	SFO_{PTV}	30.3 (27.2–33.1)	29.7 (26.9–34.5)	32.2 (29.5–35.3)	31.8 (28.4–36.5)
	SFO_{Rob}	28.5 (25.8–30.3)	27.6 (25.4–29.9)	30.6 (27.5–32.8)	29.7 (27.2–31.4)
Larynx	MFO_{PTV}	22.2 (7.0–30.3)	24.7 (13.2–32.0)	25.6 (8.2–32.7)	27.5 (14.4–34.3)
D_{mean} (Gy)	MFO_{Rob}	24.7 (7.2–31.0)	26.6 (13.6–32.6)	27.3 (8.5–33.0)	28.6 (14.9–34.7)
	SFO_{PTV}	24.6 (6.8–32.1)	27.4 (13.2–32.9)	28.1 (8.4–34.9)	29.9 (15.1–35.9)
	SFO_{Rob}	25.2 (7.8–32.9)	27.9 (14.8–34.4)	27.9 (9.5–35.3)	29.9 (16.6–36.4)
Oral mucosa	MFO_{PTV}	8.8 (5.5–28.4)	8.7 (5.3–27.9)	9.8 (6.1–31.2)	9.9 (5.8–30.5)
D_{mean} (Gy)	MFO_{Rob}	9.2 (4.4–29.0)	9.1 (4.3–28.8)	9.9 (5.1–31.1)	9.8 (4.7–30.2)
	SFO_{PTV}	8.8 (6.0–31.3)	9.0 (5.8–30.6)	10.0 (6.9–33.9)	10.2 (6.4–32.6)
	SFO_{Rob}	8.6 (5.2–31.8)	8.6 (5.1–31.1)	9.9 (6.2–33.2)	9.8 (5.6–32.7)
Constrictor muscles	MFO_{PTV}	26.5 (21.0–36.3)	26.1 (21.0–38.4)	28.8 (22.5–38.0)	28.5 (22.8–39.9)
D_{mean} (Gy)	MFO_{Rob}	26.9 (19.5–37.2)	26.3 (19.5–36.9)	28.4 (21.0–38.6)	27.8 (20.9–38.3)
	SFO_{PTV}	28.1 (20.2–37.7)	27.8 (20.9–38.7)	30.4 (21.9–40.6)	30.2 (22.6–40.6)
	SFO_{Rob}	27.7 (19.8–37.0)	27.3 (20.4–38.0)	29.8 (21.4–38.9)	29.5 (22.0–39.6)

(Continued on next page)

Table A.2. (Continued)

ROI and Metric	Plan	Nominal dose D_{Nom}		Cumulative dose D_{Cum}		Perturbed dose D_{PerNom}		Perturbed dose D_{PerCum}	
Esophageal inlet muscle	MFO_{PTV}	26.8	(2.4–29.2)	26.7	(2.5–37.0)	29.1	(3.7–32.4)	29.1	(3.6–39.2)
D_{mean} (Gy)	MFO_{Rob}	25.9	(3.1–31.2)	25.8	(3.0–36.4)	27.9	(3.9–33.7)	28.0	(3.8–38.3)
	SFO_{PTV}	26.7	(1.8–27.3)	26.1	(1.9–35.5)	29.3	(2.5–31.7)	29.1	(2.5–38.3)
	SFO_{Rob}	25.2	(3.0–31.4)	24.8	(3.0–37.0)	27.0	(3.8–34.0)	27.3	(3.7–38.8)

Abbreviations: ROI, region of interest; CTV, clinical target volume; $D_{98\%}$, dose to the 98% of the volume; $D_{2\%}$, dose to the 2% of the volume; D_{1cc}, minimum dose to the 1 cm^3 of the volume; D_{median}, median dose; D_{mean}, mean dose.

B Supplementary Material for the Bilateral HNSCC Study

Table B.1. CTV $D_{98\%}$ statistics of nominal, weekly and total cumulative doses of each bilateral HNSCC planing approach; median (range) for the cohort of 20 patients.

ROI and Metric	Dose	PTVb	cRO	aRO
Low-risk CTV	Nominal	99.3 (97.7–99.9)	98.2 (96.6–99.2)	97.5 (95.2–98.8)
$D_{98\%}$ (%)	Week 1	98.2 (88.9–99.9)	97.9 (93.8–99.4)	97.6 (95.8–99.0)
	Week 2	95.5 (79.8–100.0)	96.9 (90.2–99.1)	97.7 (96.0–99.2)
	Week 3	95.1 (82.5–99.5)	96.7 (92.8–99.1)	97.8 (95.9–99.2)
	Week 4	95.5 (83.7–99.1)	96.6 (93.8–99.1)	97.5 (96.0–99.1)
	Week 5	95.3 (82.8–99.1)	96.6 (93.5–99.1)	97.4 (95.9–99.1)
	Week 6	94.9 (82.3–99.4)	96.3 (92.6–99.1)	97.3 (94.3–99.1)
	Cumulative	94.6 (80.8–99.1)	96.1 (88.4–99.1)	97.2 (92.4–99.0)
High-risk CTV	Nominal	98.7 (98.2–99.5)	97.9 (96.8–98.8)	97.4 (95.4–98.5)
$D_{98\%}$ (%)	Week 1	97.4 (89.8–99.1)	97.8 (94.8–98.7)	97.7 (95.5–98.7)
	Week 2	95.5 (83.3–98.9)	97.6 (91.4–98.7)	97.9 (95.7–98.9)
	Week 3	96.1 (83.7–98.9)	97.7 (89.4–98.8)	98.2 (96.3–99.0)
	Week 4	95.4 (83.3–98.7)	97.7 (89.2–98.7)	98.1 (96.3–99.0)
	Week 5	96.0 (83.7–98.6)	97.6 (89.2–98.7)	98.0 (96.6–98.9)
	Week 6	95.4 (83.7–98.4)	96.8 (89.2–98.8)	97.8 (95.7–98.6)
	Cumulative	95.0 (84.5–98.5)	96.9 (89.2–98.9)	97.7 (94.2–98.6)

Abbreviations: ROI, region of interest; PTVb, PTV-based plan; cRO, classical robustly optimized plan; aRO, anatomical robustly optimized plan; CTV, clinical target volume; $D_{98\%}$, dose to the 98% of the volume.

Table B.2. CTV and OAR dose statistics for the PTV-based bilateral HNSCC plan approach; median (range) for the cohort of 20 patients.

ROI	Metric		Nominal dose		Cumulative dose	
Low-risk CTV	$D_{98\%}$	(%)	99.3	(97.7–99.9)	94.6	(80.8–99.1)
	$D_{2\%}$	(%)	113.2	(107.8–115.7)	112.2	(107.1–117.7)
High-risk CTV	$D_{98\%}$	(%)	98.7	(98.2–99.5)	95.0	(84.5–98.5)
	$D_{2\%}$	(%)	102.6	(100.7–104.8)	103.7	(99.6–111.7)
Spinal cord	D_{1cc}	(Gy)	26.4	(11.2–35.2)	27.8	(11.3–35.5)
Brainstem	D_{1cc}	(Gy)	11.9	(0.4–26.0)	12.9	(0.4–26.8)
Ipsilateral parotid gland	D_{mean}	(Gy)	23.3	(19.8–58.2)	24.8	(20.6–59.2)
Contralateral parotid gland	D_{mean}	(Gy)	20.2	(18.7–22.3)	19.9	(17.3–24.6)
Larynx	D_{mean}	(Gy)	37.9	(24.9–70.1)	39.6	(25.5–68.8)
Oral mucosa	D_{mean}	(Gy)	39.5	(17.1–66.5)	39.6	(19.6–66.2)
Constrictor muscles	D_{mean}	(Gy)	51.7	(40.3–65.5)	51.7	(38.5–66.4)
Esophageal inlet muscle	D_{mean}	(Gy)	38.4	(15.1–69.3)	39.5	(12.4–68.0)

Abbreviations: ROI, region of interest; CTV, clinical target volume; $D_{98\%}$, dose to the 98% of the volume; $D_{2\%}$, dose to the 2% of the volume, D_{1cc}, minimum dose to the 1 cm^3 of the volume; D_{mean}, mean dose.

Table B.3. Total width of the CTV $D_{98\%}$ parameter from the set of 30 bilateral HNSCC integral-treatment perturbed doses; median (range) for the cohort of 20 patients.

ROI and Metric	Plan	Total width	
Low-risk CTV	cRO	1.5	(0.5–5.5)
$D_{98\%}$ (%)	aRO	1.0	(0.2–2.9)
High-risk CTV	cRO	1.0	(0.2–3.9)
$D_{98\%}$ (%)	aRO	0.6	(0.2–3.3)

Abbreviations: ROI, region of interest; CTV, clinical target volume; cRO; classical robustly optimized plan; aRO, anatomical robustly optimized plan.

Table B.4. Dose statistics for the robust bilateral HNSCC plan approaches; median (range) for the cohort of 20 patients. The perturbed doses correspond to the worst-case values considering a range error of 0% (D_{Per0}) and a range error of ±3.5% (D_{PerR})

ROI and Metric	Plan	Nominal dose D_{Nom}		Cumulative dose D_{Cum}		Perturbed dose D_{Per0}		Perturbed dose D_{PerR}	
Low-risk CTV	cRO	98.2	(96.6–99.3)	96.1	(88.4–99.1)	95.6	(87.2–98.8)	95.2	(86.1–98.6)
$D_{98\%}$ (%)	aRO	97.5	(95.2–98.8)	97.2	(92.4–99.0)	96.6	(91.5–98.9)	96.4	(90.6–98.6)
Low-risk CTV	cRO	107.1	(104.7–110.0)	107.4	(104.5–109.0)	107.2	(104.6–108.4)	107.3	(104.7–109.0)
$D_{2\%}$ (%)	aRO	107.6	(103.6–110.8)	107.3	(103.4–109.3)	107.1	(103.3–108.8)	107.2	(103.5–109.1)
High-risk CTV	cRO	97.9	(96.8–98.8)	96.9	(89.2–98.9)	96.3	(88.7–98.7)	96.0	(87.2–98.5)
$D_{98\%}$ (%)	aRO	97.4	(95.4–98.5)	97.7	(94.2–98.6)	97.5	(93.9–98.6)	97.2	(93.8–98.5)
High-risk CTV	cRO	103.9	(102.0– 105.5)	103.5	(101.5–106.7)	103.4	(101.4–106.1)	103.5	(101.6–106.5)
$D_{2\%}$ (%)	aRO	103.9	(100.6–105.9)	103.5	(100.6–106.0)	103.3	(100.5–106.0)	103.4	(100.5–106.0)
Spinal Cord	cRO	24.9	(11.8–31.4)	26.2	(11.4–31.9)	27.0	(11.7–32.1)	27.2	(11.8–32.5)
D_{1cc} (Gy)	aRO	23.8	(12.0–33.2)	24.5	(11.2–32.8)	25.4	(11.5–32.8)	25.7	(11.6–33.0)
Brainstem	cRO	12.4	(0.4–22.9)	12.3	(0.4–24.0)	12.5	(0.4–25.2)	12.7	(0.4–25.2)
D_{1cc} (Gy)	aRO	11.5	(0.7–23.4)	11.8	(0.8–23.7)	12.4	(0.8–24.6)	12.9	(0.8–25.3)
Ipsilateral parotid gland	cRO	21.2	(19.2–55.2)	23.1	(19.2–56.8)	23.4	(19.1–57.1)	23.6	(19.3–57.1)
D_{mean} (Gy)	aRO	21.0	(16.7–54.4)	21.7	(17.8–55.6)	22.3	(18.4–56.1)	22.5	(18.7–56.1)
Contralateral parotid gland	cRO	20.0	(17.1–21.4)	19.9	(16.3–25.5)	20.6	(17.3–26.5)	20.8	(17.4–26.9)
D_{mean} (Gy)	aRO	20.0	(10.8–21.3)	19.8	(10.6–23.3)	20.5	(10.7–24.1)	20.7	(10.8–24.7)
Larynx	cRO	36.6	(23.7–69.9)	40.1	(26.9–69.8)	40.4	(27.1–69.8)	40.8	(27.7–69.9)
D_{mean} (Gy)	aRO	35.3	(24.3–69.8)	40.1	(27.1–69.9)	40.5	(27.1–69.9)	41.3	(27.7–70.0)

(Continued on next page)

Table B.4. (Continued)

ROI and Metric	Plan	Nominal dose D_{Nom}		Cumulative dose D_{Cum}		Perturbed dose D_{Per0}		Perturbed dose D_{PerR}	
Oral mucosa	cRO	38.7	(17.2–65.4)	39.6	(19.6–65.4)	39.9	(19.9–65.6)	41.0	(20.4–65.8)
D_{mean} (Gy)	aRO	40.0	(17.5–65.3)	40.0	(19.3–65.4)	40.3	(19.6–65.7)	41.1	(20.2–65.8)
Constrictor muscles	cRO	50.6	(39.4–64.4)	50.1	(39.5–63.6)	50.2	(39.7–64.0)	50.8	(40.3–64.1)
D_{mean} (Gy)	aRO	50.9	(40.3–64.4)	50.8	(40.2–63.8)	51.1	(40.5–64.3)	51.5	(40.9–64.5)
Esophageal inlet muscle	cRO	38.2	(16.2–69.7)	39.4	(13.6–66.3)	40.1	(14.3–66.3)	40.9	(14.6–66.4)
D_{mean} (Gy)	aRO	38.5	(21.8–69.3)	40.0	(16.8–70.2)	40.7	(17.2–70.2)	41.7	(18.2–70.4)
Healthy tissue	cRO	104.7	(66.4–133.3)	104.2	(67.2–131.0)	104.4	(67.2–131.1)	106.5	(68.3–134.1)
Integral dose (Gy·L)	aRO	112.8	(68.8–146.1)	112.8	(70.1–144.2)	112.9	(70.1–144.2)	114.7	(71.1–147.5)

Abbreviations: ROI, region of interest; CTV, clinical target volume; cRO, classical robustly optimized plan; aRO, anatomical robustly optimized plan; $D_{98\%}$, dose to the 98% of the volume; $D_{2\%}$, dose to the 2% of the volume; D_{1cc}, minimum dose to the 1 cm^3 of the volume; D_{mean}, mean dose.

www.ingramcontent.com/pod-product-compliance
Lightning Source LLC
LaVergne TN
LVHW041130150826
845673LV00007B/2265

* 9 7 8 3 3 8 4 2 3 0 3 0 0 *